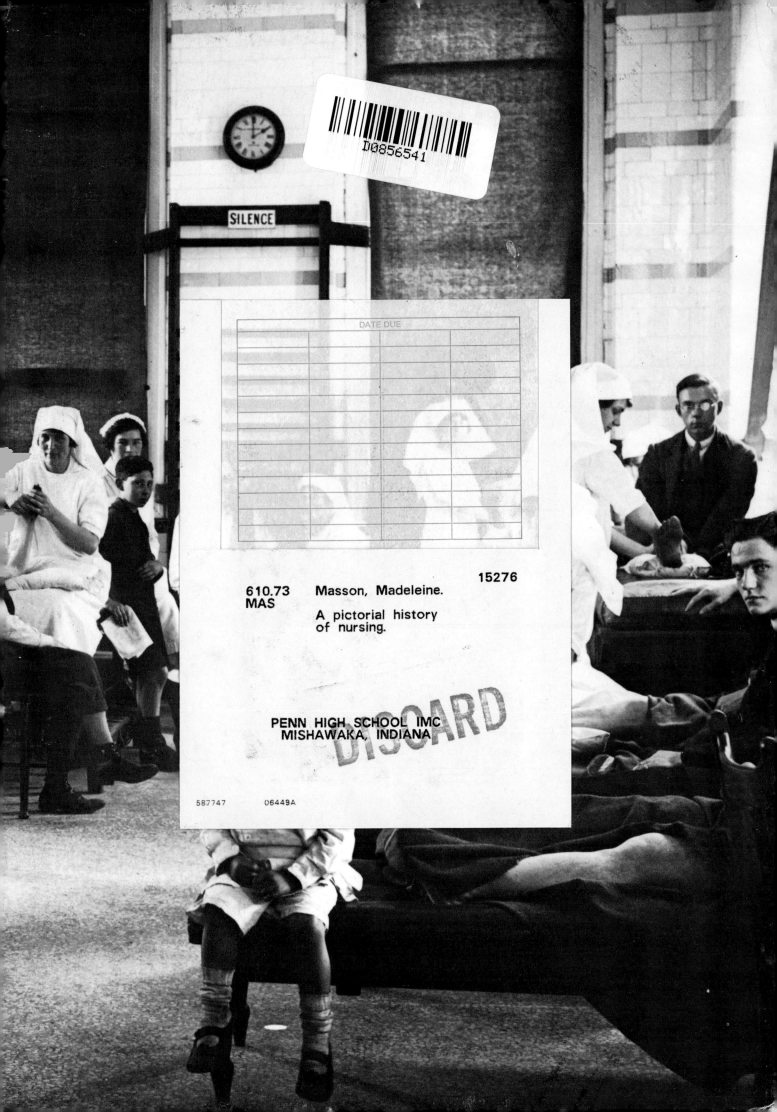

SILENCE

A Pictorial History of
NURSING

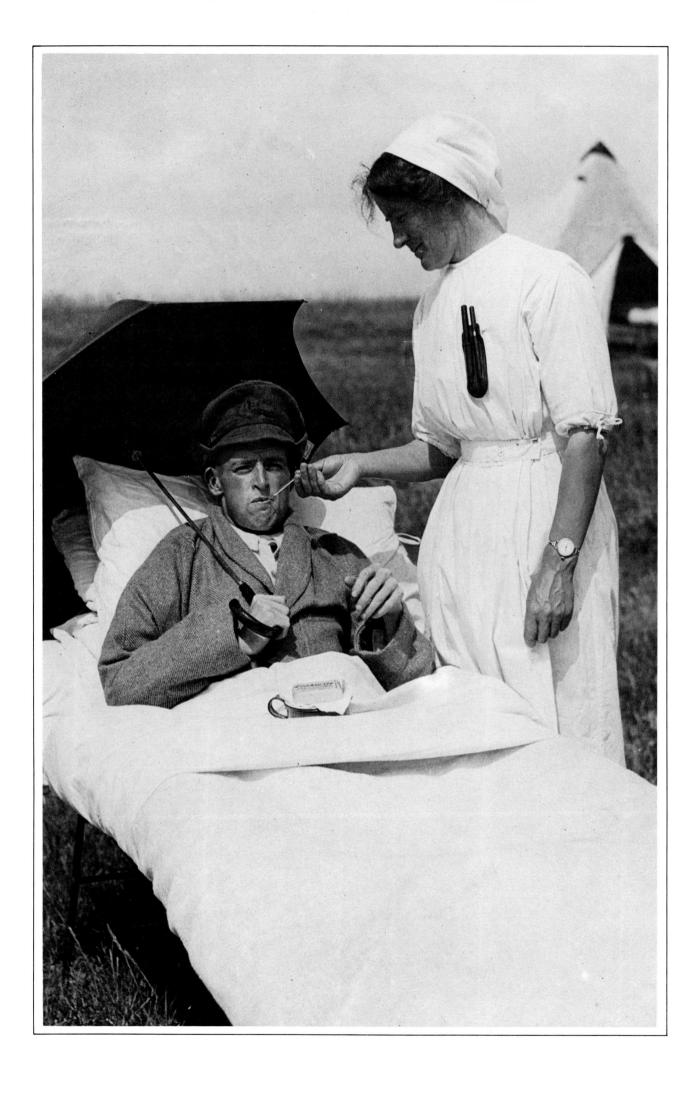

A Pictorial History of

NURSING

Madeleine Masson

HAMLYN

For Louise Frances Taber
with gratitude

Front cover 'Nurse, wounded soldier and child.' Design for a
poster by W. Hatherell, 1915.
Back cover Baby in an incubator.
Endpapers Out-patients receiving treatment at St
Bartholomew's Hospital in the 1920s.
Frontispiece A sister on active service during the First World
War takes the temperature of a wounded soldier.

Published 1985 by Hamlyn Publishing
a division of The Hamlyn Publishing Group Limited
Bridge House, London Road,
Twickenham, Middlesex.

ISBN 0 600 50062 4

Printed and bound by Graficromo s.a., Cordoba, Spain

Contents

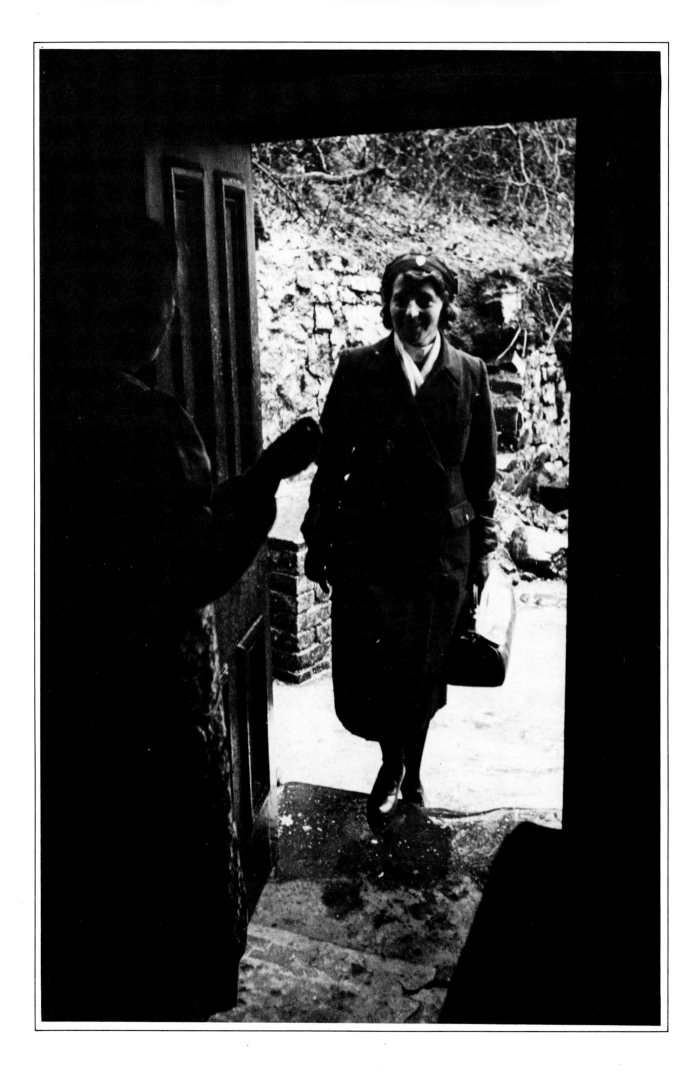

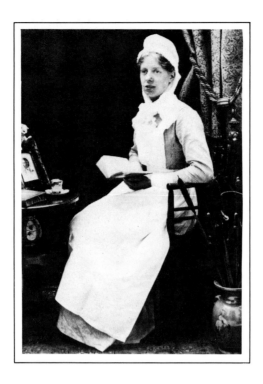

Introduction

'To tend a sick person is to pray'
Saint Vincent de Paul

The history of nursing is also the history of countless human beings who, besides being dedicated to their calling, were and are ordinary, fallible people subject to the day-to-day pressures of ordinary life. Nurses, like ourselves, have family problems, illnesses, broken love affairs, difficult marriages, problem children and crippling financial difficulties. Like the rest of us, they have to pay their bills and their taxes.

Nurses are subject to many pressures apart from those they meet in their work. Human relationships are never simple, complicated as they are by motivations which may stem from any number of sources – a power complex, a minor personality disorder, poor health, or neuroses which date back to childhood.

No matter how high the ideals of a community working together for the common good, there is bound to be friction, for not every nurse has the vision, authority, heroism or selflessness of a Florence Nightingale, an Edith Cavell or a Mother Teresa.

Yet, in compiling this history of nursing, in which I have tried to explore every aspect of this particular field to be found in person-to-person interviews, dry-as-dust reports, letters, diaries, photographs, albums and newspaper clippings, one fact emerges like a great beacon shining across the centuries and illuminating the whole canvas of nursing in peace and war. That is that nursing brings out all that is generous, unselfish, dedicated and deeply caring in those who have adopted the profession of healing and of helping the young, the old, the handicapped, the wounded and the dying.

Above *Portrait of a nurse in the late Victorian period.*
Opposite *Always a welcome sight, the district nurse arrives at the front door on her daily round in wartime Britain.*

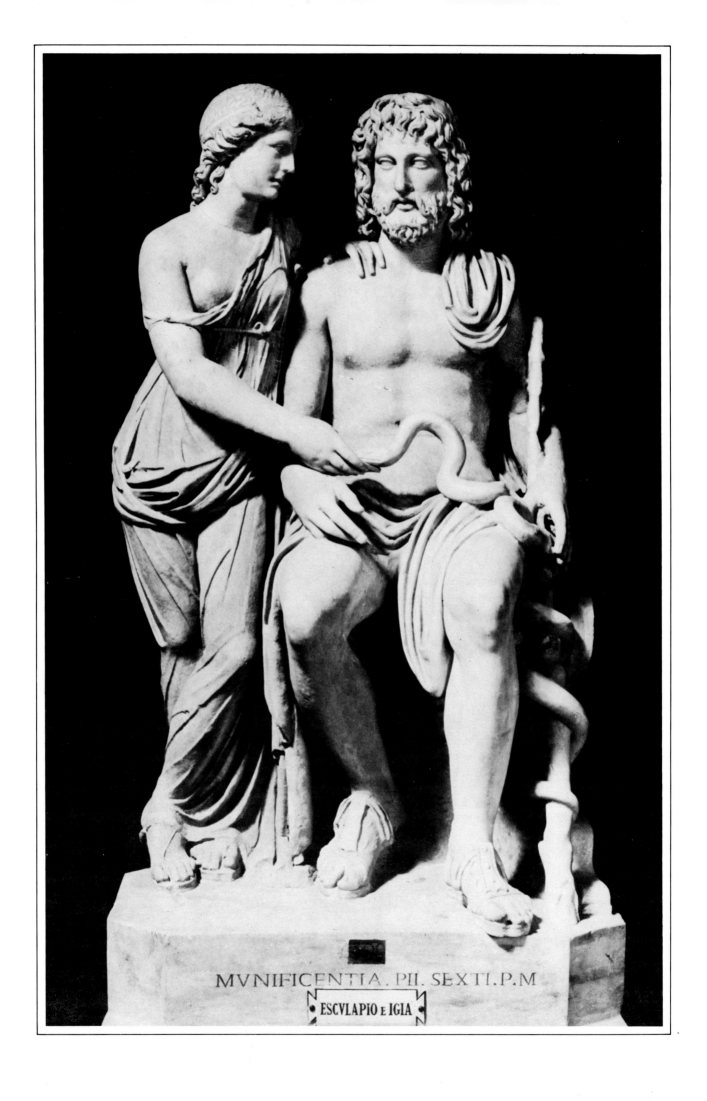

MVNIFICENTIA. PII. SEXTI. P.M

ESCVLAPIO E IGIA

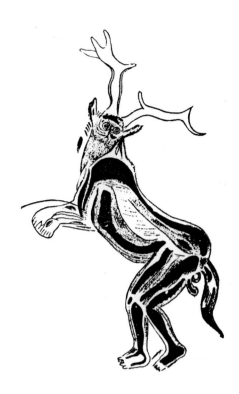

In the beginning...

Primitive medicine

Since the beginning of time illness has been part of the human condition and man has had to deal with it within the compass of his knowledge and his culture. Even before the art of writing had evolved, men and women were practising the healing arts. Primitive man's attitude to sickness was conditioned by three factors. He was unwell because a foreign body inside him was causing him pain and discomfort; he had angered his deities who were thus venting their displeasure on him; or his enemies had found an insidious way of disposing of him.

In order to rid himself of the cause of his ailment, primitive man had to turn to someone who had mysterious powers, a man who, through his superior knowledge, was in league with the unseen, and could communicate and bargain with the dark powers on his behalf. Thus did the shaman or medicine man come into being. Coexisting with him was his female counterpart, who acted as midwife, nurse and wise woman. It was she who picked and prepared herbal concoctions, made grass plasters, applied spiders' webs to sores, and

sucked and licked wounds. Through the ages there have been as many remedies as there have been illnesses, but faith, hope and commonsense generally have effected more cures than all the 'magic' devised by the shaman.

From the beginning, the instinct of the female has been to protect, comfort and nourish, and the arms that hold a baby encircle all suffering humanity, for love in the service of others is the link forming part of the long chain of healing that stretches from the mists of time to today. Man's first nurse was his mother, a warm, loving presence symbolizing security, food and warmth, and the word 'nurse' has a simple and noble origin, deriving as it does from the verb to nourish.

In the history of medicine and nursing, although the latter did not become a recognized profession until the nineteenth century, is encapsulated the history of great social and economic upheavals and of man's unending struggle to keep at bay the last enemy, death. In the history of medicine and nursing, too, are reflected elements of the great riptides of thought and discovery which, through the centuries, have brought relief and enlightenment to the afflicted in mind and body.

Top *A painting on the walls of a grotto in Ariège, France, made by a Cro-Magnon artist some 20,000 to 30,000 years ago. It depicts a medicine man wearing a reindeer skin and antlers.*
Opposite *An antique statue of Asclepius, the Greek god of healing. The son of Apollo, he is seen here with his staff and sacred snake, tended by his daughter Hygeia, the goddess of health. His cult, widespread in ancient Greece, was later brought to Rome. Vatican Museum, Rome.*

Early civilizations

Until the twentieth century it had been believed that the Greeks were the founders of scientific medicine, but we now know that other great civilizations, such as appeared in Mesopotamia, Egypt, India and China, had also built up a sound body of advanced medical knowledge. The Code of Hammurabi, inscribed on a pillar and set up in the Temple at Babylon, represented a society with well-developed laws of property and a comparatively enlightened attitude towards women. It also contained the first historical codification of medicine, and established both the fees payable to physicians for satisfactory services and the penalties, should their ministrations prove harmful. According to Herodotus' *History of Ancient Babylon*, medical care was completed by laying the sick in the public square so that any passers-by might offer helpful advice if they had had the disease or had known anyone suffering from it. Prescriptions and remedies were freely discussed and prescribed by the laity.

Evolving from a dim Neolithic culture, Egypt under the pharaohs knew an astonishing civilization which included a caste of scribes from whom eventually would come the first physicians. The arts of healing were also practised by a number of queens of Egypt, among the best known being Mentuhotep (2300 B.C.), Hatsheput (1500 B.C.), and Cleopatra (100 B.C.).

In Sumeria, Assyria, Egypt, and Greece, until approximately the third millennium B.C., the practice of healing was almost exclusively in the hands of priestesses. Yet, although midwifery was conducted only by women, priestesses did not as a rule attend confinements. Nevertheless, midwifery was early recognized as an important craft, and Sumerian midwives were given special training and education. This also obtained in the case of Egyptian midwives: the Ebers papyrus, which also offers guidance on midwifery, is based on a remarkable understanding of certain aspects of gynaecology, childbirth, abortion, breast cancer and prolapse of the womb.

The earliest known pharmacists were two Mesopotamian women of the thirteenth century B.C. but, by the end of the fourth century A.D., women had completely lost their monopoly over medicine. At an early stage the arts of healing were taken over by the male gods from the goddesses, Ea being chosen by the Assyrians and Ptah by the Egyptians. Later, when the Egyptian queen Nicrotis appointed Imhotep as the first court physician, she started a new cult in which men superseded women in all medical matters. Imhotep was not slow to make the most of his opportunities, became the patron of doctors and was finally elevated to the rank of god, thus joining Ptah. Later, the Greeks were to identify him with Asclepius, their own god of healing.

Besides amulets and talismans, the Egyptians used at least one-third of all medical substances known to us today. These included opium, gentian, castor oil and colchicum (used for gout). Therapy was based on diet, enemas, the external application of animal fat, and also purging and bleeding, which remained the main resources of physicians until well into the nineteenth century.

In India, in the third century B.C., under the inspired leadership of the emperor Asoka, hospitals were built, which may have been the first examples of state medicine, staffed by doctors and nurses paid for by the government. The

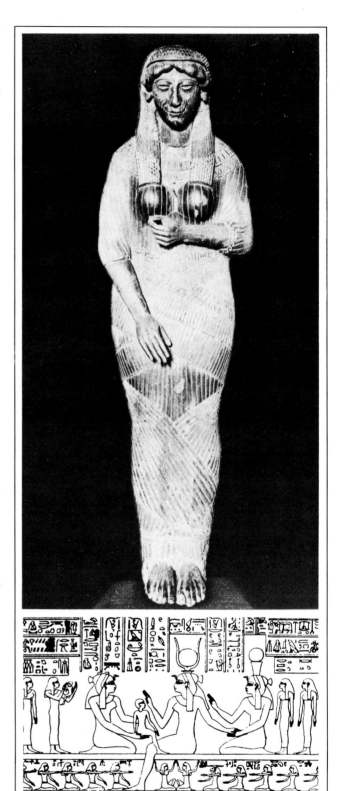

Top *Hathor, the Egyptian goddess who gave assistance to women in childbirth. Wood sculpture from Memphis.*
Above *A nurse holds a newborn infant in front of the goddess mother, Isis. From a decoration in the Temple of Dendera, Egypt.*

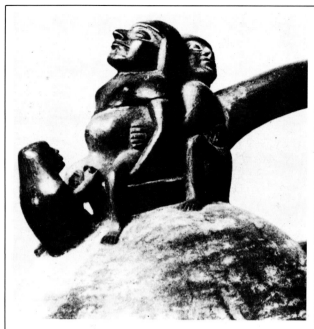

An Inca vase depicting the delivery of a child. Museum für Völkerkunde, Berlin.

Caring for the sick was thought to be part of the normal domestic duties of the female. Her main function was to bring children into the world and, when necessary, find her a substitute or wet-nurse. The Book of Exodus in the Old Testament recounts how Moses' sister asked Pharaoh's daughter, 'Shall I go and call thee a nurse of the Hebrew women to suckle your child?'.

The Jews, though scrupulous in regard to cleanliness and general hygiene and possessing sound dietary laws, looked upon any human knowledge of healing with disfavour, since they thought it was a power that should belong to God alone. Few remedies are mentioned in the Old Testament, though Naaman the Leper was told by Elisha to wash himself seven times in the River Jordan, while King Hezekiah, 'sick unto death' from a boil or abscess, was bidden by Elijah to apply a lump of figs to the afflicted part of his body.

Midwives had their part to play in Biblical days, and birth stools or obstetric chairs are specifically mentioned as being part of the ritual of birth, as are two midwives named Puah and Shiprah.

nurses were male, hand-picked for their special qualities, and had to comply with hospital rules which stated that the nurse should be skilled and reliable, and able to do anything which the patient's condition required.

In ancient China, which was to develop a civilization far in advance of that of any western country until the Middle Ages, great importance was attached to colour in the treatment of illness. Red, the colour of blood, was always associated with healing. Mummies were painted with red ochre to restore a life-like appearance. Red flannel was worn around the neck to prevent sore throats, and a red thread wound about the neck and tied with nine knots was thought to be sovereign against nose-bleeds. The Chinese also discovered and used many drugs, ranging from ephidrine to camphor. They practised acupuncture, moxibustion (cauterization by means of moxa), and inoculation against smallpox. The Emperor Shen Nung, who lived around 300 B.C., was the father of Chinese medicine. His *Pen Tsao* or *Great Herbal*, contained over 1000 drugs, many of which are still in use today.

Women and healing

While nursing and medicine have always been interrelated the medical profession ignored the merits and usefulness of the great body of devoted, though untrained, women who laid out bodies, birthed babies, prepared meals, and quietly went about the many menial tasks demanded by the condition of the sick. Not until the advent of Christianity was there any recognition of nursing as a separate occupation.

Greek medicine

About 2000 B.C. a mixed body of invaders swept into the Greek peninsula and islands and the western regions of Asia Minor. Here they established one of the most extraordinary civilizations of all time. The famed medical system that they developed originated in Asia Minor, and spread throughout the Greek world. Its roots are veiled in legend, in which healing and religion are mingled. Apollo, the sun god, was also god of health and medicine. He was supposed to have been born on the island of Delos which was both a shrine and a medical centre. Apollo, it was said, taught the art of healing and of medicine to the centaur Chiron, who in turn instructed Jason, Achilles and Asclepius. The last-named instructed his sons in medicine, and they, according to the poet Homer, tended the Greek armies at the siege of Troy.

By the mid-eighth century B.C. Asclepius had become the Greek god of healing with, as his symbol, a sacred snake. He had two daughters, Panacea, and Hygeia, who was goddess of health. The sanctuaries of Asclepius were renowned through Greek history as places of healing, and in the greatest of them all, at Epidauros, the sick slept in porticos 'beyond the temple', as is described by Pausanias about A.D. 175. The ruins of these, now excavated, are thought to have been the earliest known example of a hospital ward.

Although women were excluded from medical schools and from temple practice, they continued to play an important part in healing, at home, among the poor and among women. They prescribed herbal treatments, but their main value in the eyes of the Greeks was as midwives. The 'obstetrix' was present at most births and could also procure abortions when the need arose. The mother of Socrates was said to be a skilled midwife.

About the fourth century B.C. a woman called Agnodice, wearing men's clothing and with her hair cut short, was accused of practising medicine under false pretences. She was brought to trial, but the clamour raised by the women of Athens, who demanded her freedom, saved her from punishment.

The inscription on the pedestal of the statue of Antiochis, a Greek woman doctor of the first century B.C., states that she was honoured by the city authorities 'for her practical skill in the medical art'. Two centuries later, Galen spoke of a 'salve of Antiochis for sufferers of the spleen, from lumbago, dropsy and arthritis'.

In 460 B.C. one of the greatest figures in medicine, Hippocrates, was born at Cos. He was the first teacher in history to assert that disease was not due to the actions of demons but to neglect of natural laws, and was to be explained on physical grounds alone. Hippocrates demanded the highest moral and ethical standards of the physician, and the Hippocratic oath which bears his name is still in use today.

It seems clear from the writings of Plutarch and Xenophon that it was the duty of the wife to nurse not only her family but her slaves. 'Whenever a slave is sick,' says Ischomachus to his young wife, 'you must look after him.' Plutarch mentions 'an old serving dame' who waited on a sick man.

The contribution of Rome and early Christianity

It was due to the Roman genius for organization that hospitals for the sick and wounded – military hospitals – were first founded. We know from inscriptions that doctors were attached to the army and the navy. They did not rank as officers, but had certain privileges. It is thought that the Emperor Augustus first created this particular medical service when the army became permanently established in camps.

The philosopher Seneca alludes to the 'valetudinarium of a rich house' and to the slave 'to whom in a large household has fallen the task of keeping under control the sick and the demented.' Columella in his De Rustica, writing of the duties of an overseer, says: 'If, as it so often happens, a slave is wounded at his work, and is injured thereby, he is to have poultices applied. Should another be ill, he is to be taken immediately to the valetudinarium where the overseer will order the correct treatment he will need.'

In another passage it is laid down that the overseer's wife is to take care of the health of the slaves, and to keep a special watch out for malingerers. It is also her duty to look after the valetudinarium and keep it clean, in good order and ready to receive new patients at all times.

Seneca says that there were valetudinaria in the imperial household, which may well have been staffed by specially trained male and female slaves who carried out the orders of the imperial physicians. If Seneca was correct, these slaves –

male and female – would have been the first trained nurses (midwives were in a category of their own) in history.

Several Roman military hospitals, built about A.D. 100, have been excavated in the Rhine and Danube valleys. They were probably used as base hospitals for frontier forces. The ground plans reveal long corridors opening into a series of suites. In addition, there were central courts for kitchens, dining-rooms, pharmacies, etc. There were no open wards, so it may be assumed that each soldier-patient enjoyed a degree of privacy. It is also reasonable to suppose that either slaves or soldier-orderlies staffed these military hospitals, a type of service which would be customary in military hospitals until Florence Nightingale went to the Crimea.

While it is generally believed that before the Christian era accommodation was provided for the aged and sick in places of refuge which were later to become almshouses and hospices, it was not until the spread of Christianity that the sick were treated with more care and consideration, and that the more repellent aspects of nursing were ennobled by a sense of devotion to a great cause.

Those most active in such services were the women of the new faith. St Paul in his Epistle to the Romans wrote: 'I commend to you Phoebe our sister, which is a servant of the Church for she hath been a succourer of many, and of myself also.'

The first hospital is thought to have been founded by St Basil of Caesarea, about A.D. 350, while, according to St Jerome, who died in 420, the first hospital to be built in Rome was financed by a wealthy woman called the Lady Fabiola. She was one of the first of a long line of dedicated women to renounce a life of ease in order to devote themselves to nursing the sick. Fabiola may have been one of the first of the deaconesses, the women who adopted the Greek word diakonein, which means 'to serve or to minister', as their motto. There were deacons as well as deaconesses, men who ministered to the sick in the monastery hospitals where no women were permitted to enter.

The Arabs, who contributed notably to early surgical techniques, had a hospital in Baghdad in the tenth century. A little later the staff employed in a hospital in Cairo are specifically stated to have included both male and female nurses.

History is starred with the names of noble people who gave their lives to nursing. Among them are St Radegund of Poitiers and St Hildegarde of Bingen on the Rhine. St Radegund, the daughter of one French king and the wife of another, left her sadistic husband and founded a great convent of which she became the abbess. Here she nursed the sick and lepers until her death in A.D. 589. The name of St Hildegarde ranks as one of the foremost in the annals of nursing. Besides being one of the most brilliant scholars of her time, she devoted herself to the care of the sick who came to her convent. Some centuries later a Byzantine princess, Anna Commena (1083–1148), a historian, wrote of her experiences when she took charge of a large hospital in Constantinople in time of war.

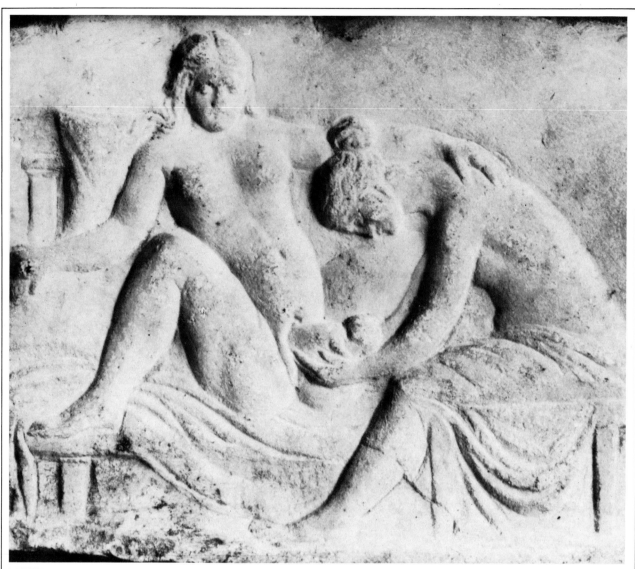

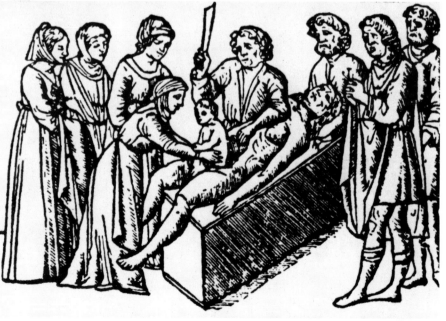

Above *A Roman bas relief showing a child being delivered.* **Left** *An illustration from a sixteenth-century edition of the works of Suetonius depicting the birth of Julius Caesar by Caesarean section. In fact, contrary to popular belief, Caesar was not born in this way.*

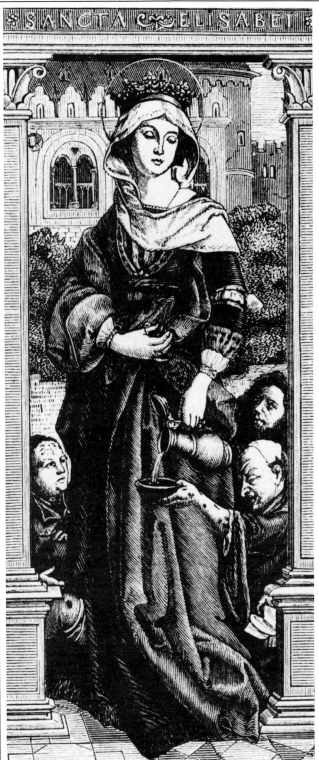

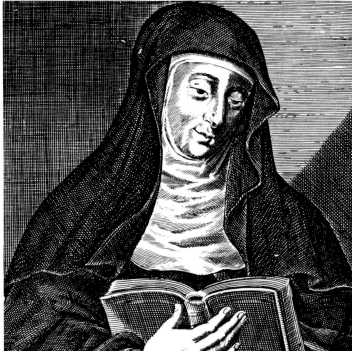

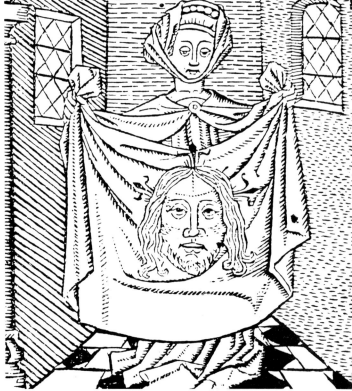

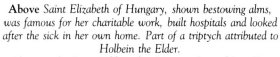

Above *Saint Elizabeth of Hungary, shown bestowing alms, was famous for her charitable work, built hospitals and looked after the sick in her own home. Part of a triptych attributed to Holbein the Elder.*
Above right *Saint Hildegarde of Bingen devoted herself to the care of sick people at her convent.*

Above *Saint Veronica who, according to tradition, lent her veil to Christ on his way to the cross to wipe his brow. With this veil she reputedly cured people suffering from various diseases and was also known for her work among lepers. Woodcut, 1482.*
Opposite *Saint Radegund of Poitiers, a sixth-century queen of France, who founded a convent in which she nursed the sick and lepers.*

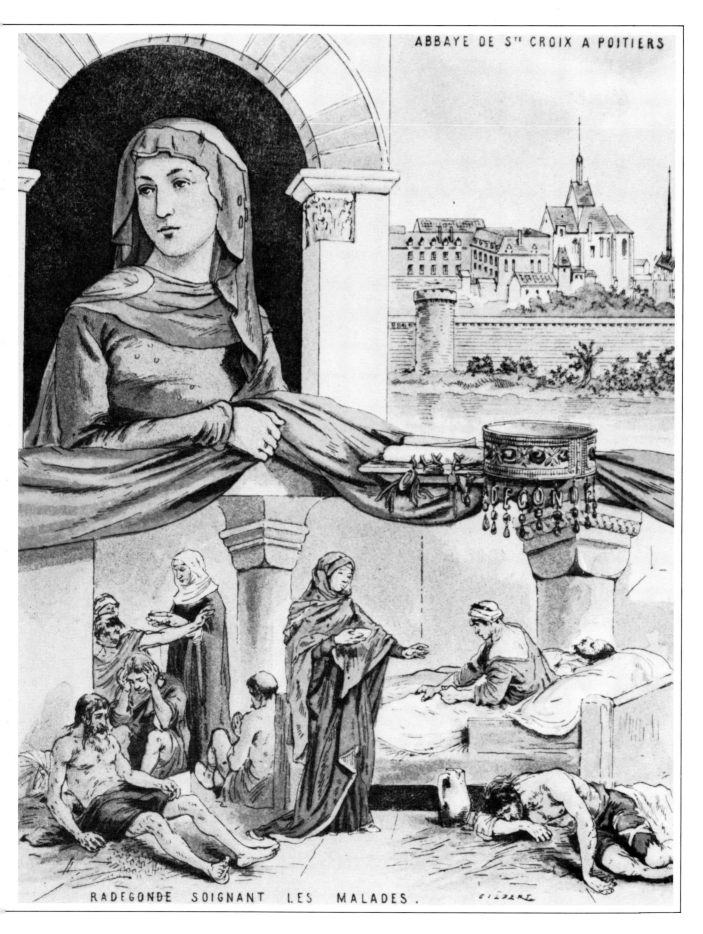

ABBAYE DE Sᵗᵉ CROIX A POITIERS

RADEGONDE SOIGNANT LES MALADES.

GILBERT

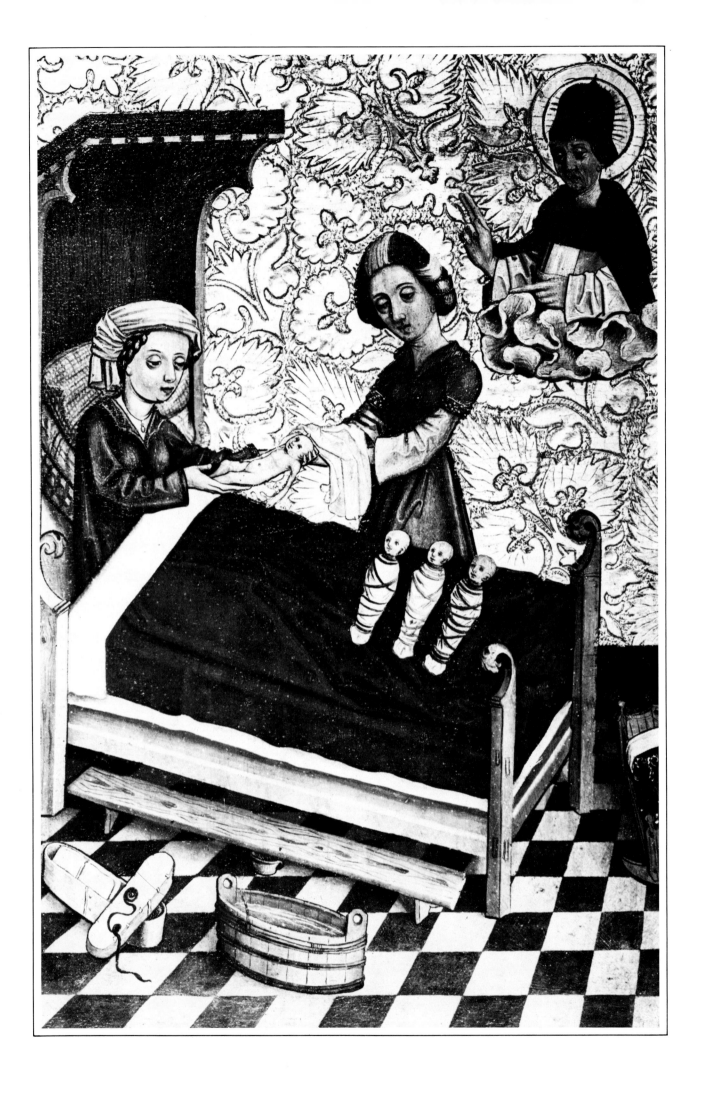

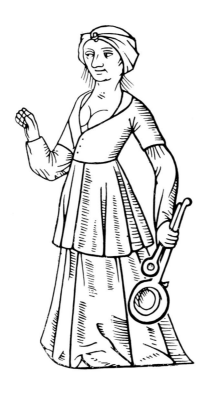

Nursing in the Middle Ages: hospitals, midwifery and plague

Hospices, hospitals and military orders

The constant flow of travellers and pilgrims brought the first hospices into being. The hospice, from the Latin *hospitium* (place of entertainment), became a house of shelter for travellers in dangerous countries. The earliest and best known hospices are those in the Swiss Alps, instituted possibly for the sake of the pilgrims travelling to and from Rome, and retained by monastic orders.

The Great St Bernard Hospice, founded in 962, is noted for its help given to travellers stranded in the snow or overtaken by cold, and for the breed of dogs specially trained for rescue work. Others are the St Gotthard, started in the thirteenth century, the Simplon, the Little St Bernard, and one on Mt Cenis.

The name hospice was subsequently extended to homes for the destitute and sick. However, the era of the hospital proper may be said to have begun in the twelfth century, when a distinction was made between refuges intended for

sick persons and institutions intended to house the aged and infirm. As the care of these people was supposed to be a religious duty rather than a responsibility of the civil authorities, the building and direction of hospitals was in the hands of the Church. The hospital was thus an ecclesiastical, rather than a medical, establishment and skill and science were judged to be less effective than devoted care, allied to religious and spiritual concerns.

Almost simultaneously with the new concept of the hospital (St Bartholomew's Hospital, Smithfield, was founded in 1123 and St Thomas' Hospital in southeast London, in 1200), there emerged from the earlier monastic system various orders, both religious and secular, whose main duty was to nurse and care for the afflicted. These included military nursing orders, some of which were the outcome of the Crusades, notably the Knights Hospitallers, the order today represented by the Order of St John of Jerusalem, whose duty was to care for pilgrims and the sick. Their birthplace was the celebrated hospital built by Justinian in Jerusalem 100 years after that established by the Lady Fabiola in Rome. The Knights grew in riches and power, and the lavish equipment and efficient management of their hospitals were a source of envy to all. There was also a woman's branch of the Order formed by the Lady Alix (Agnes) in Jerusalem, who became the head of the female community. After the Muslim reconquest of Palestine, the nuns fled to Europe, to Spain, where, under the patronage of

Top *A nurse carrying a candle saucepan. Fifteenth-century French woodcut.*
Opposite *Mother with quadruplets. In medieval Europe expectant women were generally safer in the hands of midwives than they were with doctors. Fifteenth-century Tyrolean painting.*

Queen Sancha, wife of Alfonso II, they established a convent at Sigena in Aragon in 1188.

Other famous military orders formed at the same time were the Knights Templar, the Teutonic Knights (who combined military with nursing duties), and the Knights of St Lazarus, who devoted themselves entirely to the care and nursing of lepers.

Regular and secular orders

One of the oldest and most famous of the regular orders was that of the Augustinian Sisters of the Hôtel Dieu of Paris. By the thirteenth century they were formed into a strictly monastic community under the rule of St Augustine. Both the hospital and the community were governed by the clergy. The most complete records of medieval hospital administration are those of the Hôtel Dieu. Built near the Cathedral of Notre Dame, in the thirteenth century the hospital already had five wards, and worked according to an elaborate system. It was ruled by a prior, under episcopal authority, with a prioress in charge of the sisters who did most of the actual nursing. The novices did all the washing, mostly on the banks of the Seine. By modern standards conditions in the hospital were far from perfect, indeed insanitary. Since space was at a premium the sick lay six or more to a bed, their linen was infrequently changed and liberal doses of small ale or wine took the place of nourishing foods or vitamin-filled fruit. But the sisters were devout, humane and patient, and did their best for the miserable specimens of humanity in their care.

The secular orders, so called to distinguish them from the knightly orders and regular communities with perpetual vows, made great progress in the early thirteenth century. These were lay members of religious orders, men and women who, though they did not live in a community, wore the habit and took part in the works of some great order. Their growing importance was attributed to the spread of the Franciscan order, and especially to that most famous of all secular branches, the Third Order of St Francis (whose members are known as Tertiaries).

Yet another secular order was that of the Béguines, which was founded in 1180 in Belgium. Its members were women

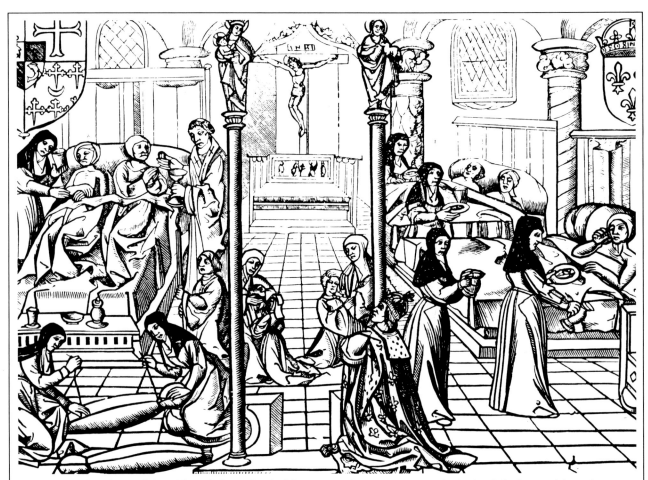

A ward in the Hôtel Dieu Hospital, Paris. On the left a priest and a nun minister to the dead and the dying, while in the foreground nuns are sewing shrouds. On the right is a more cheerful scene, with patients taking nourishment. Sixteenth-century wood engraving from a Manuscript Register in the Burgundy Library, Brussels.

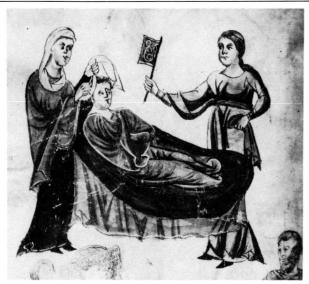

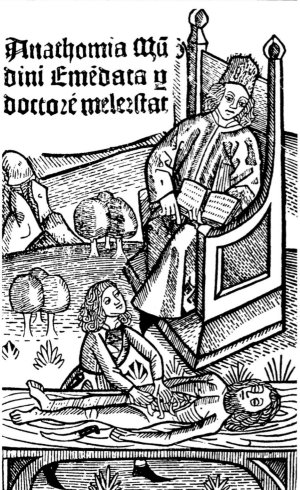

** Anathomia Mū dini Emēdata p doctozé melezstar**

Top *Two nurses attending a bedridden patient. Thirteenth-century manuscript. Oesterreichische Nationalbibliothek, Vienna.*
Above *A dissection by a female assistant under the direction of Mondino de' Luzzi, the great Italian medieval anatomist. Woodcut frontispiece from Mondino's* Anathomia, *published at Leipzig c. 1493.*

who lived in communities in small houses in an enclosed precinct in the shadow of a church or hospital.

Finally, there was domestic nursing. This was thought to be the concern of the female members of families, who nursed not only their ailing relatives but their domestic staff as well. Many women at that time had a knowledge of herbs, cordials and traditional remedies and, under the supervision of physicians, gave their patients simultaneously purges and emetics.

The role of women in medicine and midwifery

To escape the generally subordinate position of women in society some of the more determined sought to acquire fulfilment and a life outside marriage and the family circle. Their options were limited, but a number succeeded in establishing notable careers in regular communities of nuns. There were even joint monasteries, housing men and women living in separate establishments, but ruled over by a woman superior. Many women chose to become midwives, while others sought to practise medicine. Women had in fact been permitted to become doctors until the sixteenth century when they were disbarred from the medical profession, and were severely persecuted if they made any attempt to trespass on what was considered to be exclusively male territory.

Until that time women students were made welcome at the famous medical school at Salerno in Italy. Founded in the ninth century, it reached its apogee in the twelfth, and kept its great lustre and fame until the end of the fourteenth. Towards this centre flowed all the great currents of medical thought, ancient and contemporary, and it naturally attracted large numbers of brilliant young medical students.

Among the most famous was Trotula, whose name appears on the lists of those practising medicine in the eleventh century. According to one source she lived at Salerno about the time of the last Lombard prince and was celebrated as *sapiens matrona* and *mulier sapientissima*. The book that bears her name, *De passionibus mulierum*, a treatise on obstetrics, may have been a later compilation of her material. Among others things it gives sound advice about the choice of a wet-nurse and the specific diet she should follow. It is interesting to note that Trotula is mentioned in Chaucer's *Canterbury Tales* under the name of Dame Trot.

It would appear that throughout medieval times medical men had no skills to offer to expectant women equal to those provided by a midwife. The earliest textbook on the subject was *Die Schwagern Frauen und Hebammen Rosengarten*, written in 1513 by Eucharius Roesslin at the request of Catharina, Duchess of Brunswick, to help pregnant women and midwives, and translated into English in 1540 as *The Byrthe of Mankynde*. Roesslin was not impressed with the capacities of the average midwife. In a scathing comment he wrote:

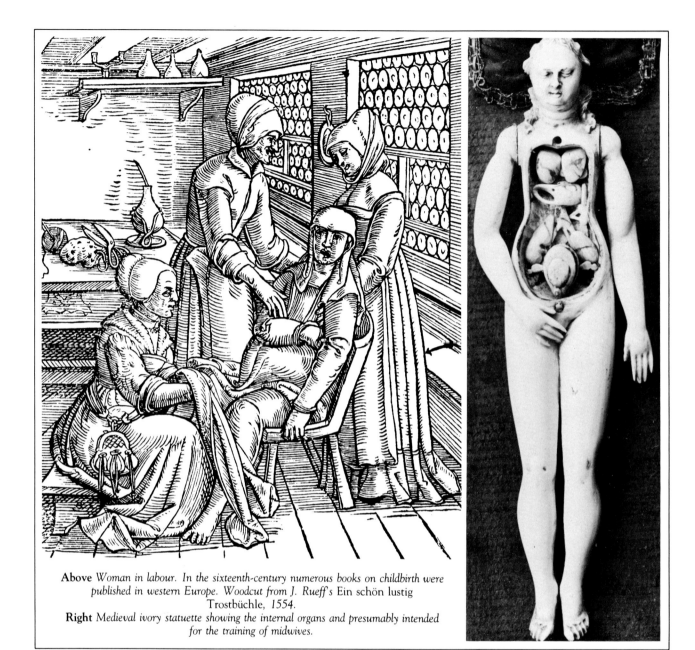

Above *Woman in labour. In the sixteenth-century numerous books on childbirth were published in western Europe. Woodcut from J. Rueff's* Ein schön lustig Trostbüchle, *1554.*
Right *Medieval ivory statuette showing the internal organs and presumably intended for the training of midwives.*

I'm talking about the midwives all
Whose heads are empty as a hall
And through their dreadful negligence
Cause babies' deaths devoid of sense.

The truth about the work of midwives lay somewhere in between the ferocious indictment of Roesslin and the more complimentary remarks made by women whose lives, and those of their babies, had been saved by the ministrations of their local midwives.

Most of these were elderly women who practised their trade in small country towns and villages. They could hardly be called qualified, in our sense of the word, but they were practical and experienced, most of them having borne many children. The fact that they were ignorant, illiterate and superstitious, relying greatly on folklore and folk remedies and were often thought to be witches, did not diminish their usefulness or the importance of their role in society.

Many works on obstetrics intended for women were published in the sixteenth century in France, England and Germany, but these made little contribution to the improvement of hygiene in the labour room. This was generally crammed with friends and relations while the unhappy mother-to-be groaned, sweated and pushed, or screamed as she was prodded and torn with crude and cruel obstetric instruments which differed little from those used in ancient times.

It was not until 1574 that the first manual on nursing was published. Its author, Jacob Oetheus, put forward sensible views, stressing the importance of following the orders of the physician and recommending the employment of married men and older women as nurses.

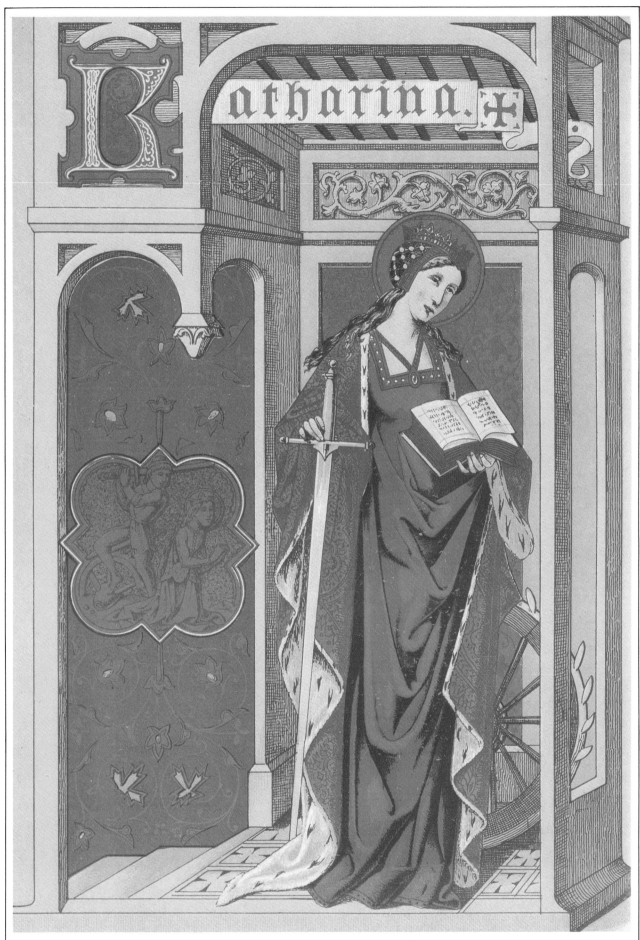

Saint Catherine of Siena, noted for her visions, revelations and devotional works, was also associated with nursing and the care of the sick.

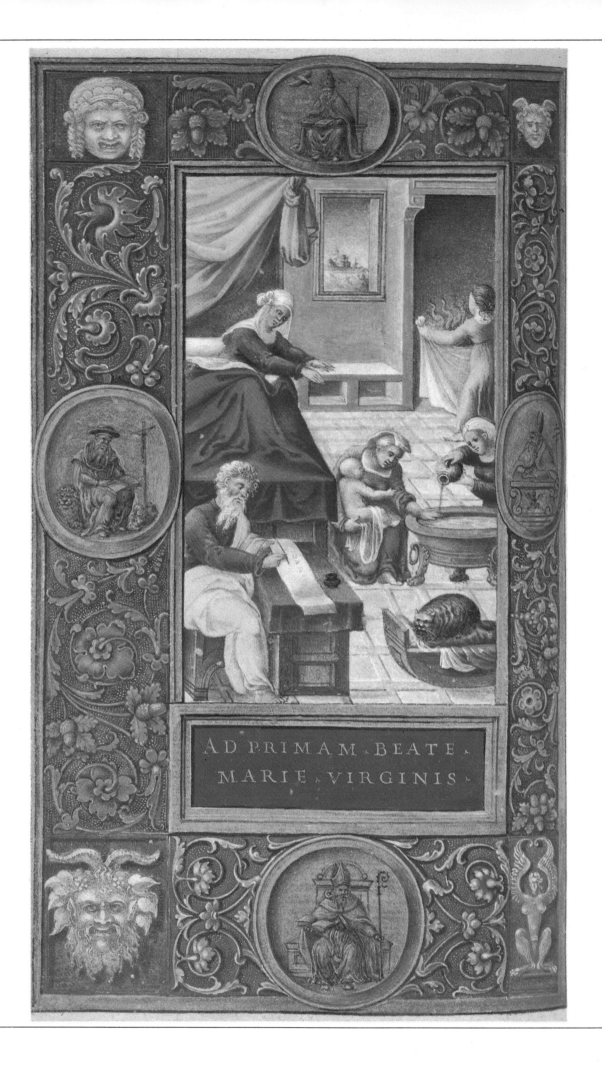

AD PRIMAM BEATE
MARIE VIRGINIS

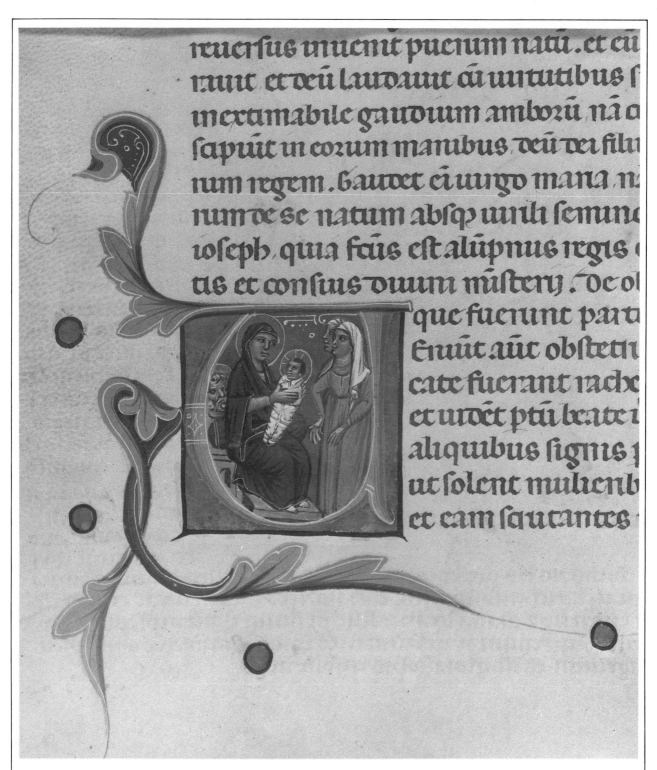

reuerfus inuenit puerum natu. et eu
...ruit. et deu laudauit cu uirtutibus f
inextimabile gaudium amboru na o
sapuit in eorum manibus. deu dei filu
rum regem. Gaudet ci uirgo maria n...
...rum de se natum absqp uirili seminc
iofeph. quia frus est alumpnus regis ...
...tis et consius diuim misterij. De ol...
...que fuerunt part...
...Enuit aut obstetri...
cate fuerant rache...
...et uidet ptu beate i...
aliquibus signis ...
ut solent mulierib...
et eam scrutantes ...

Above *Two midwives at the birth of Christ. Acts of St Mary*
and Jesus. Fourteenth-century Italian manuscript.
Opposite *Birth of St John the Baptist. Zachariah writes at a*
table while midwives prepare a bath for the baby. Sixteenth-
century Italian Book of Hours.

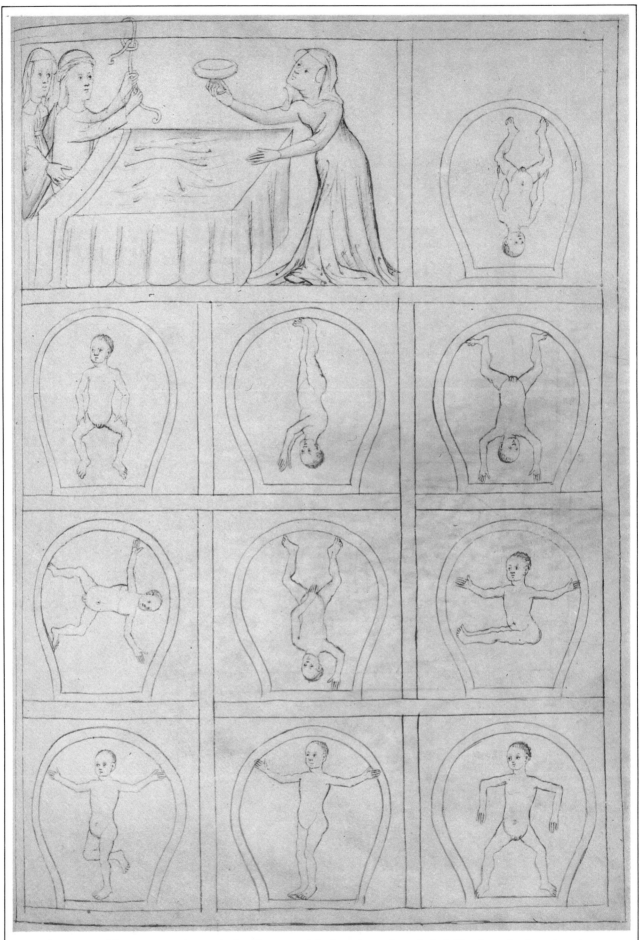

A woman in labour supported by a midwife pulls on a cord fixed to a beam above the bed. Drawings of embryos in various positions. Medieval English manuscript.

Leprosy and plague

Life in medieval and Renaissance Europe was a hazardous business. Living conditions were primitive and life-expectancy at birth was low. Infants and young people were mostly undernourished, suffered from ailments such as rickets and scrofula, and rapidly succumbed to almost any infection. Insane persons generally had short shrift, for many were believed to have sold their souls to the devil in return for magical powers. Local beldames thought to be witches were immediately blamed if any disaster threatened the community in which they lived. Such disasters were many and various, but two of the greatest scourges of medieval times were leprosy and the Black Death or bubonic plague.

Leprosy has been known from time immemorial. It is frequently referred to in Egyptian papyrus and stone records. It was prevalent in India and China, and was believed to have been brought from the East by the Crusaders. Sufferers from the disease were compelled to wear a distinctive yellow dress and to carry a bell or clapper. This they rang at intervals, crying out as they approached towns or villages, 'unclean, unclean!' They were forbidden to enter churches, but might watch the service through a hole in the outer walls known as the leper's squint.

The majority of lepers were rounded up and lived in common misery in special settlements known as lazarettos. The afflicted were cared for mainly by the Knights of St Lazarus. There were also Sisters of St Lazarus, for the Bull of Pope Urban VIII in 1262 confirmed the privileges of the order for both sexes.

Leper houses were built all over Europe and are estimated to have numbered 19,000 in the thirteenth century. Many compassionate royal personages – mainly women – did all they could to make the plight of the lepers a little easier. Queen Matilda, wife of Henry I of England, built a hospital at St Giles-in-the Fields in London, and in both London and the provinces there were many places of refuge for the lepers, the first of which was founded at Rochester about 1100.

As early as 1346 rumours reached Europe of an unidentified disease which was ravaging China and India. Travellers returning from these far places spoke of the terrible death suffered by those stricken by the malady. Nobody thought it would reach Europe, but it did, brought by ship along the trade routes. Carried through Armenia to the entrepôt stations of the Italian merchants in the Crimea, it spread like wildfire among the Tartars, eventually arriving in an Italian seaport in the spring of 1348.

Reports of the horrors of the bubonic plague soon reached the remotest corners of Europe. It was infectious to the last degree and it spared its victims no physical humiliations, for it enveloped the sufferer in a revolting stench.

The medical faculty had no idea as to the cause of the plague. They attributed its ravages to a number of factors including 'corruption of the atmosphere', the movement of the stars, a judgment from heaven and changes in the

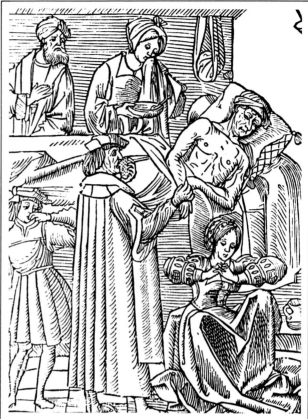

A plague victim attended by a physician holding a sponge to his nose both as a means of protection against infection and against the smell given off by the patient. Sixteenth-century woodcut from Fasciculus Medicinae.

weather. Since over-population in Europe was the cause of many ills, including malnutrition, the peasant was the perfect target for the Black Death, and none of those who died ever knew that their end was attributable to the bacillus *Pasteurella Pestis* which lived a cosy, sheltered life in the bloodstream of an animal, or in the stomach of a flea. The flea normally favoured as a home by the bacillus chose as its residence the hair of the black rat, *rattus rattus*, and it was this wiry rodent which brought the plague to Europe.

Remedies of all kinds were tried. One of them was an amber apple, which was made with a mixture of fine soil, sieved and washed, and then macerated for seven days in a mixture of rose-water, laudanum, benjoin, storax, amber, civet and musk. After maceration the mixture was rolled into apple-sized balls. It was thought that aromatic oils and the smoke from dry and scented woods might keep the plague at bay. Anything aromatic was of value.

Having scythed its way through France, the Black Death arrived in England in 1349. It came first to Melcombe Regis (now part of Weymouth) in Dorset, carried in a ship which had sailed from Bristol. One of its crew had brought with him from Gascony a flea, *pulex irritans*, which was also a carrier of the fatal pestilence. The plague raged for over two and a half years in England, killing about one-third of the population.

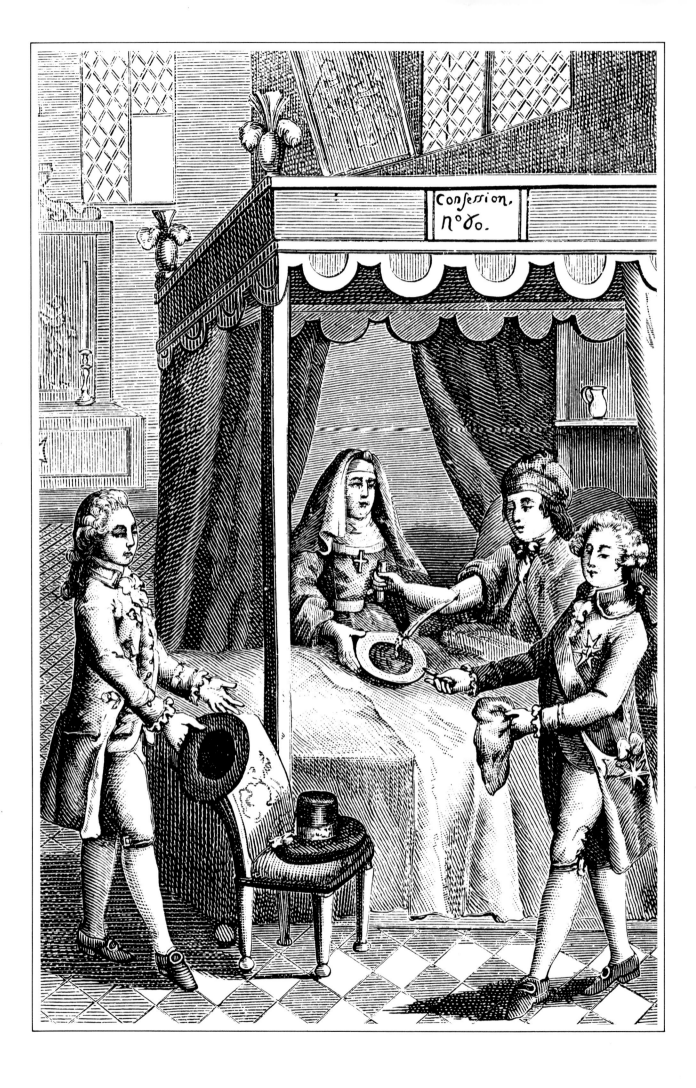

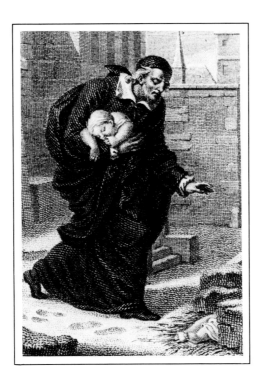

The Reformation and after

Nursing and the Reformation

The Reformation, the great religious upheaval which took place in the sixteenth century, led to the division of all Christendom and had a shattering impact on almost every aspect of life and society. In England Henry VIII determined to repudiate the authority of the papacy because it thwarted his plans to divorce his Spanish wife, Catherine of Aragon, and marry Anne Boleyn. Brushing aside all obstacles, he went on to assert his own supremacy as head of the Church of England, and then proceeded, with the assent of parliament, to the confiscation of nearly all ecclesiastical property and the complete suppression of monastic establishments (1535–7).

Since England at that time, alone of all European countries, possessed no hospital system other than that practised in the convents and monasteries, and no nursing class, the result was that the sick and the poor who had relied on the monastic system of philanthropy were left to fend for themselves as best they could.

In 1547 the City of London requested Henry VIII's son, Edward VI, to grant permission to take over the city's largest hospitals, St Bartholomew's, Bridewell, and Bethlehem, so

as to be able to house and help the afflicted. According to some historians, this move was the beginning of the poor law system, and eventually, during the reign of Elizabeth I, the first regular Poor Law was instituted by the civil government for general public relief. Thereafter, the sick poor in small towns and villages were sent to the almshouses set up by the poor law boards and supported by local taxation.

In the case of St Bartholomew's the hospital was governed by the mayor and by a self-perpetuating board of its own. In this way it did not come under the direct control of the City of London, and later served as a model for the first hospitals in the American colonies.

During the entire period of the reorganization of St Bartholomew's patients stayed in the wards. After alterations five 'sisters' were appointed to look after the patients, and the nurse in charge of these took the title of matron – one of the few monastic customs to be retained. Although the matron and nurses were lay people, it was decreed that they should continue the custom of the religious sisters by wearing a habit, which in time was to evolve into the nurse's uniform.

The directions given to the sisters of St Bartholomew's in 1544 stated that they should 'do their duty towards the poor in making of the beds and keeping clean their wards, as also in washing and purging their unclean clothes and other things'.

There were never enough sisters to care for all the sick, and servant-attendants were employed to do the rough work. By the 1600s a class of women helpers had become an ancillary arm of the nursing services in hospitals. These were simple, illiterate women who possessed a smattering of

Top *Saint Vincent de Paul rescues abandoned children in the streets of Paris. They were cared for in foundling hospitals built by him.*
Opposite *Bleeding a patient in the Hôtel Dieu Hospital, Paris. Eighteenth-century.*

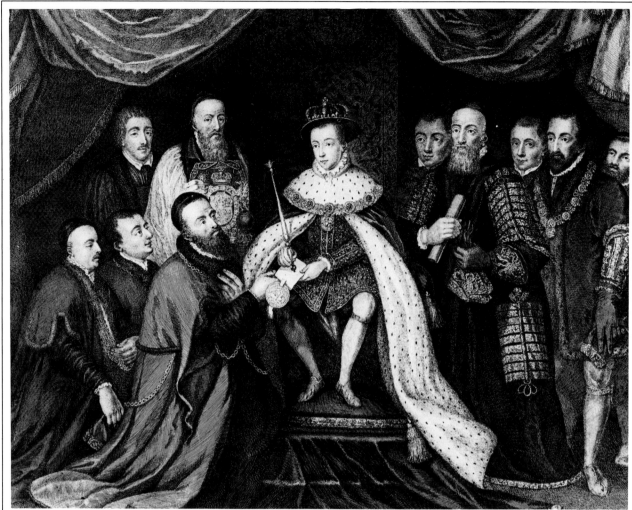

Edward VI presents charters to the three London hospitals—Christ's, Bridewell and St Thomas'—in the presence of assembled dignitaries of the City of London. From a painting by Hans Holbein.

nursing knowledge allied to experience in domestic tasks. The sisters and, to a lesser degree, the helpers, were expected to observe a discipline almost as strict as that of the nuns. However, much of the religious devotion and zeal that had inspired the nuns, who considered their work a personal service to God, no longer motivated the secular staff of the hospitals.

Since medical science at this time required no specific training for nurses, and hospital management was left in the hands of lay personnel, the standards of nursing declined, and for three centuries after the Reformation secular nursing, in England at least, was considered menial work to be done by menials.

Saint Vincent de Paul

In France the work of Saint Vincent de Paul was to prove immensely beneficial for the sick and for the future of nursing in general. Born in Gascony in 1576, this remarkable man was educated at a Franciscan college, and later earned his living as a private tutor, being ordained a priest in 1600. Captured at sea by Turkish pirates, he was sold into slavery at Tunis, but escaped back to France, where he became chaplain to Queen Marguerite de Valois.

In 1632 he founded the Daughters of Charity, the first order of uncloistered women devoting their lives to works of charity among the sick and needy. These ladies, known as Les Dames de Charité, undertook to visit the sick in their homes in order to give them nursing care and spiritual help. The first superior of the new order was a woman of noble birth, Louise de Marillac. It was she who recruited the first contingent of strong country wenches to help the Dames, the first, Marguerite Naseau, starting work in 1630.

The movement instigated by Vincent grew and diversified, and in 1654 an important development took place. The women were allowed to nurse wounded French soldiers, whereas in Britain only orderlies were permitted to nurse soldiers in military hospitals.

Hospitals in the New World

The sixteenth and seventeenth centuries witnessed the setting up of European colonies in America, thus bringing about the first contact between Europeans and Indians. However, the latter had not, in fact, waited for the arrival of the white man to find cures for their sick. Their medicine men knew the virtues of many healing plants such as cascara and chinchona bark. Nevertheless, in spite of the advanced civilization of the Mayas and Incas, there is no evidence of hospitals in Mexico or Peru.

Spain planted colonies in Central and South America, and Spanish civilization was established much as it was in the homeland. The medical science of the Renaissance was cultivated in the universities founded in Lima and Mexico City, and in them were built the first hospitals on American soil.

The first French hospital established in North America was the Hôtel Dieu in Montreal in 1665. However, the English colonists in North America, while building various types of almshouses, did not found a proper hospital until 1750, when a Doctor Thomas Bond and other Philadelphia

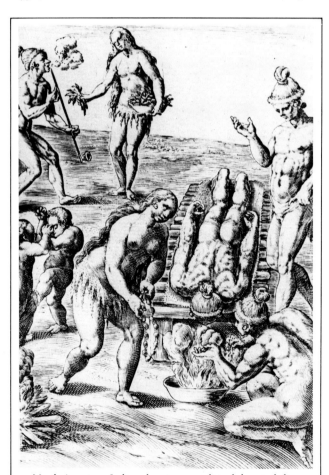

North American Indians burning a medicinal drug to help a patient suffering from a respiratory disorder. Sixteenth-century engraving by Théodore de Bry.

physicians proposed that a general hospital be set up in Pennsylvania.

Health in eighteenth-century England

England itself in the early eighteenth century was still a land of hamlets and villages. Such towns as existed were mainly on the coast. In Lancashire, the West Riding and West Midlands towns of substance were beginning to grow, but the majority of the population was still located in the south and still predominantly rural. The towns were as insanitary as their hospitals, when they had them, and houses and cellars were desperately overcrowded. Typhus, typhoid and dysentery were widespread and could easily devastate whole families. At this time only one child in four born in London survived.

The poor continued to multiply and, unlike the rats, to starve. The Elizabethan Poor Law of 1601, later modified by the Stuarts, was still operative, the parish being responsible for relief. In the 1720s the problem became too much for the parish alone to bear, and in 1723 parliament was finally obliged to enact legislation which would enable parishes to combine for the purpose of erecting a workhouse or union. These unions were then hired out to any manufacturer who, in return for keeping the inmates alive, obtained cheap labour. Nursing as such had no place in the lives of these people, who considered hospitals as the last refuge of the incurably ill and dying.

Although there were 'sisters' in both St Thomas' and St Bartholomew's hospitals in London, the general standard of hygiene and nursing in civil hospitals at this time was deplorable. Open windows and ventilation were considered dangerous. Damp seeped through the walls, mildew and fungus sprouted in corners, and cockroaches and bugs flourished. The patients were covered with lice and, since they suffered from scabies and malnutrition, they died like flies. The duties of the nurses included scrubbing, doing the laundry, and emptying spittoons and close-stools. There was an almost total lack of even the simplest equipment. Night-nursing was unknown, though the matron in some hospitals was supposed to get up twice a week in the night, and go into the wards to make certain 'that the children were covered in their beds'.

However, the history of both hospitals and of nursing was influenced by the progress of medical science and by new approaches to both health and hygiene but, while the patients profited from more expert doctoring, nursing did not. This was because, once the physicians had gained entire control of the patients, they directed every move of the nursing staff, taking away from them all authority and initiative. It was no wonder that nursing in the early eighteenth century was carried out mainly by incompetent slatterns.

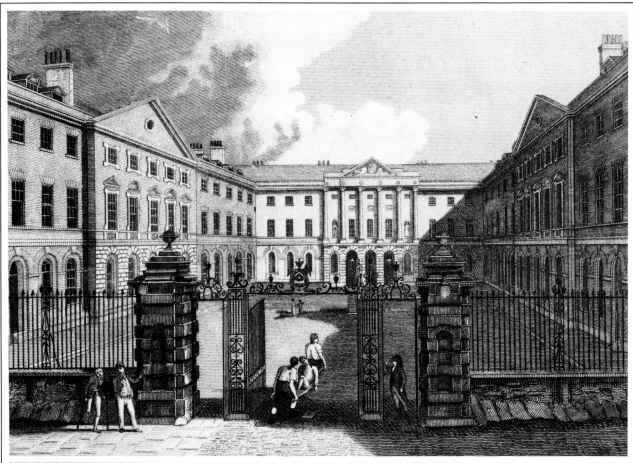

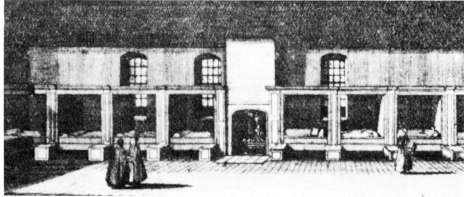

Above *The entrance to Guy's Hospital.*
Left *A ward in the hospital. Guy's was one of a number of hospitals founded in England in the eighteenth century.*

Guy's Hospital

Yet a wind of change was blowing through England, passing through the ramshackle warrens of filth, squalor and disease in which the majority of its people lived and died. Wealthy men who had made large fortunes and, for a variety of reasons, wished to assist their fellow men, began dedicating much of their wealth to founding and endowing new hospitals.

Such a man was Thomas Guy, printer, publisher and freeman of the Stationers' Company and of the City of London. He had acquired a tidy fortune through printing a vast quantity of bibles. This he invested in South Sea stock which, in his old age, suddenly increased fivefold, making him a very rich man indeed. He had always cherished the idea of being able to found a hospital, designed and built for the purpose of accommodating all its activities under one roof.

Guided by the advice of Dr Richard Mead, one of Guy's closest friends and the most famous physician of his time, the printer-philanthropist studied the plans of the architects selected to carry out his ideas. Sadly, he did not live to witness the opening of the hospital, for he died in Dec. 1724. Two years later, Guy's Hospital, with accommodation for 435 patients, opened its doors. Although the important

School of Nursing at Guy's was not formally established until 150 years later, the first reference to a nursing staff was made at a meeting of the Court of Committees in May 1725, when the 'Court elected Anne Rowney as Matron at a salary of £50 per annum.' It was also 'resolved that the salary allowed to the Sisters be £25 per annum, of which sum £5 per annum be allowed for providing crockery ware and one pair of Clean Sheets on the admission of every fresh patient (as the custome now is at the Hospital of St Thomas). . .'

When the hospital opened the nurses came in daily, their uniform being a medallion inscribed with the name of the ward and the status of the owner, which the nurses hung round their necks over their own clothes. Nurses frequently figured in the minutes of the Court of Committees as being 'drunk and disorderly'. Excerpts from the minutes of the Court from 1726 onwards show that embezzling provisions, pawning patients' clothes, drunkenness, admitting disorderly people and neglect of patients were frequent occurrences.

In 1752 the duties of the sisters and nurses were recorded as follows:

> 'That they wash or cause to be washed all weak peoples' clothes without taking money or reward for same.
>
> To attend the Surgeons during the whole time of Dressing – to stupe [place a hot compress upon] as often and in such manner all such patients as the doctor shall direct.

> To scour and make clean all bedding that be foul and to wash all foul rowlers [bandages] and rags and to see that none of the said rowlers be wasted or destroyed through her neglect.
>
> They must attend the Butler at the ringing of the Beer Bell and not suffer such patients as carry the beer to embezzle it by the way – in like manner at the ringing of the Bread Bell and also of the Cooks Bell'. *History of Nursing. Guy's Hospital 1725–1968.*

Other hospitals

By the mid-eighteenth century Britain could boast a considerable number of hospitals. In 1719 Addenbrooke's was founded at Cambridge. St George's came into being in 1734, the Edinburgh Royal Infirmary in 1736, the Rotunda Hospital, Dublin, in 1745 and St Luke's in 1751.

The Middlesex Hospital was founded as a charity for the sick and lame of Soho and the terrible slums of Seven Dials around St Giles-in-the-Fields. First known as the Middlesex Infirmary, it was accommodated in two small terrace houses in Windmill Street, off Tottenham Court Road, opening its doors in Aug. 1745. This hospital, incidentally, was financed entirely by voluntary subscriptions until the founding of the National Health Service.

The wards in the Middlesex were typical of those of most hospitals. They were long, with the beds in parallel rows.

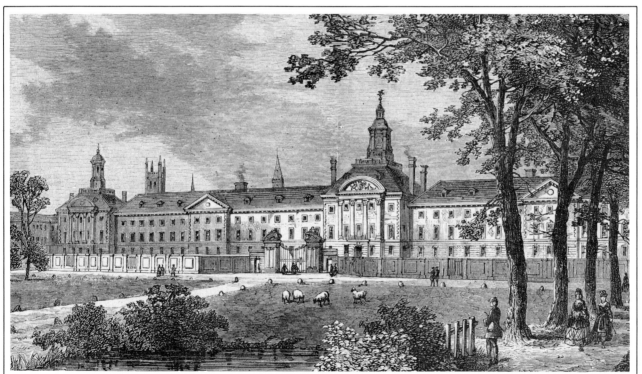

A view of Bethlem Royal Hospital (Bedlam) at Moorfields in the mid-eighteenth century.
It had been moved to this site in 1675.

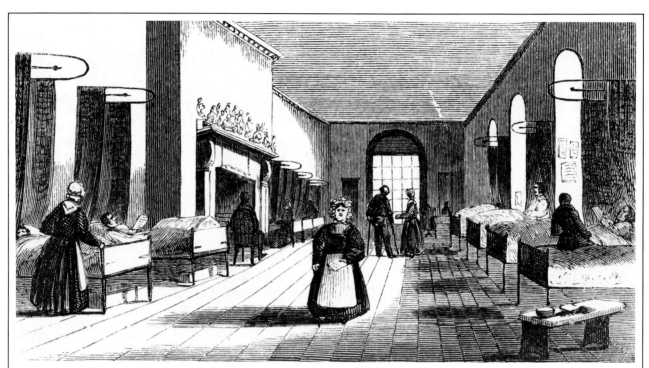

The interior of Rahere ward, St Bartholomew's Hospital, London, in the 1840s when there was already much concern about conditions in English hospitals. From An historical sketch of the priory and royal hospital of St Bartholomew *(1846).*

The bare boards were either washed or covered with sand, a process known as 'dry rubbing'. The mattresses which covered the wooden beds were stuffed with straw or hair which, in a number of hospitals, provided ready homes for bugs.

The first maternity ward in a general hospital was opened at the Middlesex in 1747. Another hospital which was to break new ground was the New Westminster Lying-in Hospital, which was to become the General Lying-in Hospital, York Road, Lambeth, in 1765. One of the objects of this hospital was to provide for the 'reception and immediate relief of indigent soldiers' and sailors' wives', the former in particular being very numerous in and about the City of Westminster. The moving spirit in the founding of this hospital was Dr John Leake, a brilliant man who dedicated himself to obstetrics and to the finding of sponsors to build his pet project, a new lying-in hospital. Leake, like Dr William Cadogan, another physician with advanced views, had revolutionary theories about the rearing of babies, and he suspected that the feeding bottles used at this time were in some measure responsible for the mortality of tiny babies in the care of foster-mothers. The feeding bottles were made of horn or earthenware and the teat of thin leather, often a glove finger with a perforation in it. Milk was put into these bottles, but more often mixed with flour and water to make a pap. Milk bought in London was generally sour as a result of bacterial action and these methods of artificial feeding were well known as causes of digestive upsets in babies. Leake also upheld Cadogan's views on the wearing of tight swaddling clothes and on diet. Cadogan suggested that children should wear loose clothing and be weaned on to fruit, vegetables and butter early in their lives.

Hospital reforms

The standards of nursing even in the great hospitals were still very low, and though intelligent and humane people like Madame Necker, wife of the minister of finance under Louis XVI, founded a hospice 'to shew the possibilities of nursing the sick in single beds', very few French hospitals followed her advice.

Another dedicated reformer was John Howard (1727–89), whose survey and observations on the many hospitals, prisons, lazarettos and places of detention he visited were to prove the greatest possible value to the nursing profession. According to Howard, most hospitals employed nurses who were in reality ignorant and illiterate domestics with little control over their patients, and who could, as at St Thomas', be out of their ward until 8 p.m. in summer and 7 p.m. in winter. Most patients supplemented their diet – thin gruel for breakfast, six ounces of meat for dinner (but no vegetables), broth for supper and a daily ration of two to three pints of beer – with liberal libations of gin procured from the numerous gin shops.

The first systematic attempt to train hospital attendants was made by Dr Valentine Seaman of the New York Hospital. As early as 1798 he organized a course of 24 lectures which included the outlines of anatomy, physiology

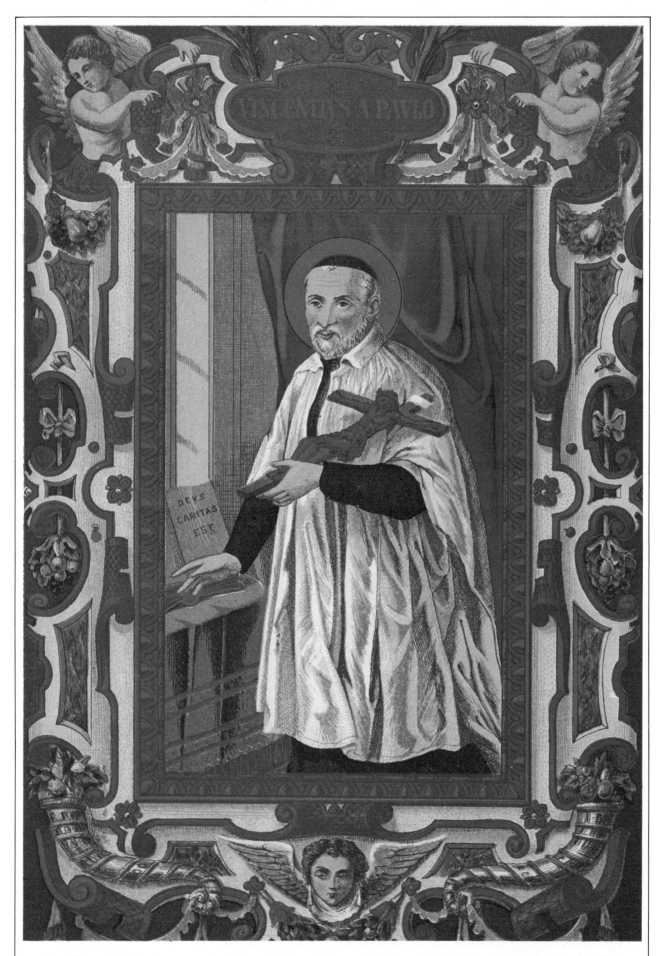

Saint Vincent de Paul, whose many charitable activities paved the way for important nursing reforms. He was canonized in 1737.

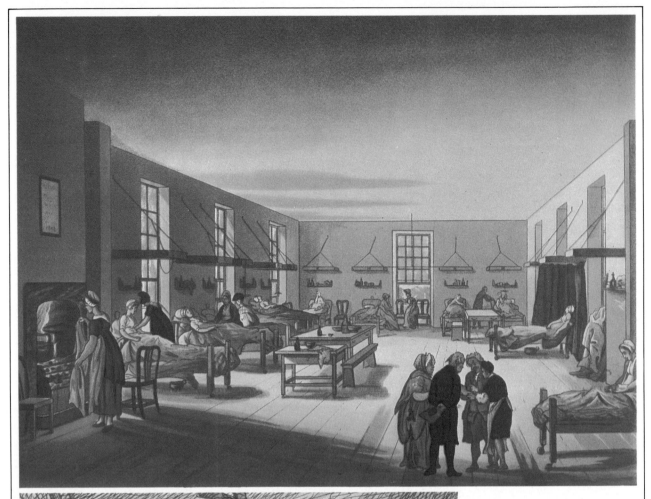

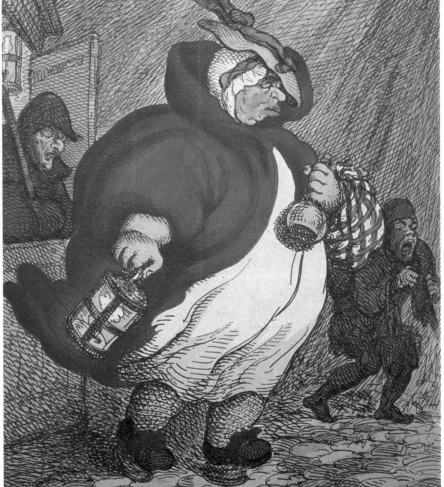

Above *The women's ward in the Middlesex Hospital, London, at the beginning of the nineteenth century. Aquatint by Stadler after a painting by Thomas Rowlandson and A. C. Pugin.*
Left *A midwife. In the early nineteenth century neither midwives nor nurses in general stood very high in public esteem. Etching by Thomas Rowlandson.*

and child care, the course being run in conjunction with the maternity department.

By the late eighteenth century specialized hospitals dealing with particular illnesses were being built. The old 'group' system, which consisted of herding patients together no matter what ailed them, changed for the better and, since hospitals, like jails, reflected social conditions in general, already in 1760 the beginnings of a hospital reform system were emerging. These also included more humane treatment of the insane, much of which was due to the efforts made by two men, an Englishman, William Tuke, and a French doctor, Philippe Pinel.

Efforts were made to introduce special nursing equipment; china and glass replaced the iron mugs and tin plates in general use. The use of oiled cloth as draw-sheets helped to keep incontinent patients cleaner. Iron beds and hair-mattresses replaced verminous pallets, and alcoves and curtains were removed to allow better ventilation in the wards.

However, it was not until the medical profession discovered that proper nursing was a vital factor in the care and recovery of their patients that any attempt was made to replace the slatternly hospital attendants by a better class of woman. Doctors also came to realize that it was important that the nursing staff under their orders should have some kind of preliminary training in providing remedial as well as custodial care.

This revolutionary new approach to nursing was expressed in an article in a French encyclopedia in 1765. The author wrote the following:

> 'This occupation is as important for humanity as its functions are low and repugnant. All persons are not adapted to it, and heads of hospitals ought to choose their nursing staff with care, for the lives of their patients may depend upon the choice of applicants.'

It was in Germany, however, that the greatest developments in nursing had taken place. Manuals on the subject had been available since the sixteenth century when the Early Christian role of the deaconesses had been revived. The deaconesses generally devoted themselves to visiting the sick poor in their community, a role which would eventually be taken over by the health visitor.

However, it was Professor Franz May of Mannheim who, horrified at the high mortality rate of babies born in hospitals, revolutionized nursing by putting forward the idea of having a nursing school attached to a hospital. He was lucky enough to have his blueprint approved by the authorities who allowed it to be advertised in the local papers.

The professor, having invited male and female hospital staff to attend his lectures, gave them detailed instruction on hygiene, diet, bleeding and bathing. He then made a further bold move, begging surgeons and physicians to try to remedy the miserable conditions in which nursing staffs lived and worked. Semi-trained, hard-worked, chivvied and on duty around the clock, they could really not be expected to give the patients the care and attention needed.

The civil authorities agreed with him, but his medical colleagues rose up in a body to protest at what they said were his efforts to undermine their authority and May had to back down, although he never ceased canvassing for better conditions for the nurses. Eventually his persistence overcame all obstacles, and between 1782 and 1815 the first nursing schools were founded in Germany. Unfortunately, however, the nursing staffs in Protestant hospitals in England and on the Continent still came from poor backgrounds, were untrained, and often given to drink and to promiscuity with their male patients.

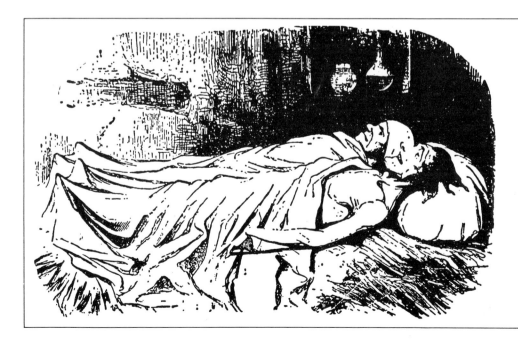

The living and the dead lying side by side in the same bed. One of the more unpleasant experiences which patients at the Hôtel Dieu Hospital in Paris had to endure at the beginning of the nineteenth century. From a lithograph by Honoré Daumier.

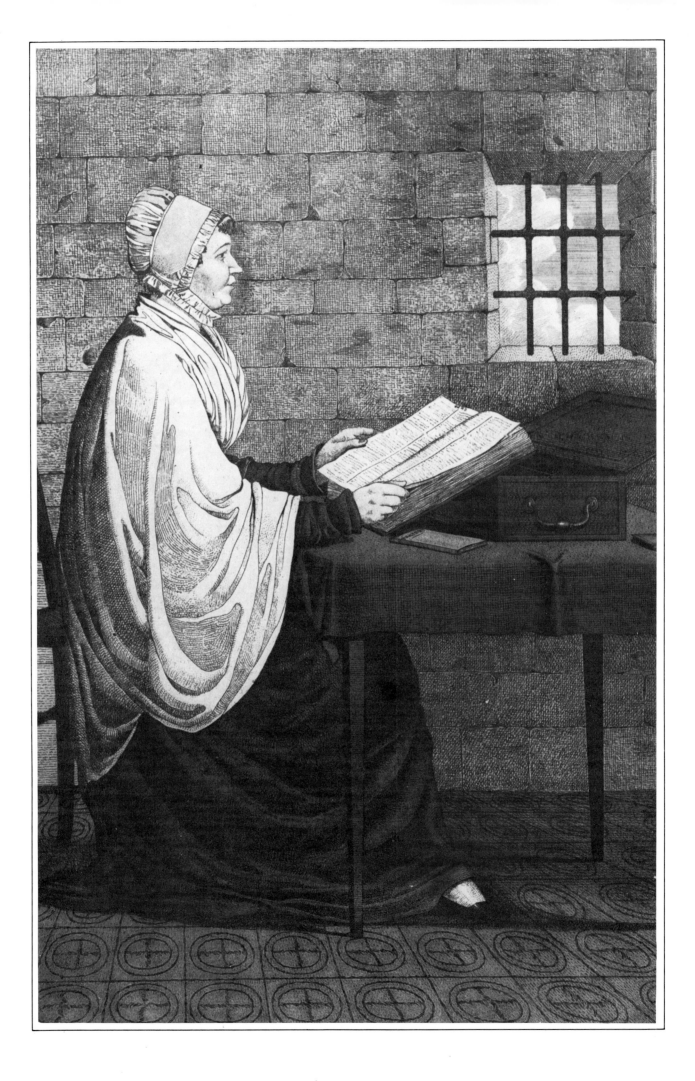

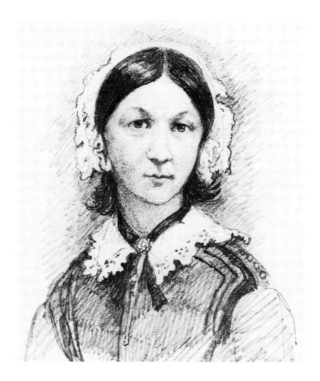

The pioneers of modern nursing

Two women who were to have a considerable influence upon the social history of their country were born within a year of each other, Queen Victoria in 1819 and Florence Nightingale in 1820. Although the circumstances of their lives were obviously very different, both became strong-willed, determined women who admired each other and were in their turn objects of veneration to their countrymen.

They came into a world of change and conflict. Britain was still recovering from the effects of its long struggle first with Revolutionary and then Napoleonic France. In the North and in the Midlands new cotton mills were built, and new blast furnaces poured out mass-produced iron, as the Industrial Revolution transformed England from an agricultural into a manufacturing nation, bringing profound changes in the lives of its people.

The changes did not at first seem to be for the better. Wealth poured into the coffers of the new industrialists, but the population appeared to be increasing at a frightening rate, adding to the misery of unemployment which the postwar depression had brought to the workers in the new industries.

Even the solid fabric of society seemed to be in danger, as were the moral values on which that society had been based. However, although the licentious tradition of the Regency was still very much in evidence it was being challenged by the new seriousness of the Evangelical movement, created by a deep religious feeling and a conviction that if society were to survive the distress and discontent of war and the postwar years, the ruling classes must set an example to the lower orders. Thus was born a new generation of humane reformers, of whom Elizabeth Fry was a pioneer.

The work of Elizabeth Fry

The daughter of a Quaker banker, John Gurney, she was brought up in surroundings of comfort and culture. She married Joseph Fry, like her father a wealthy Quaker banker, and in 1813 paid her first visit to Newgate Prison. This was her 'road to Damascus', for the filth and misery she found there determined her to devote all her energies to improving the lot of the prisoners, particularly the women.

To her dismay she discovered that there were only two rooms set apart for the sick at Newgate. Although the men's room had seven beds, the women's had none, and patients were compelled to lie on the floor. There was no professional medical care, and only after many complaints was a doctor paid to visit the sick prisoners.

Elizabeth Fry set up a school for children in the prison and helped the women prisoners to form classes in which they could learn various skills such as knitting, sewing and making patchwork quilts. Her fearless and caring approach in her relationship with the prisoners soon had an effect, and her methods were followed and copied by enlightened people all over Europe.

Top *Florence Nightingale.*
Sketch by G. Scharf, 1857.
Opposite *Elizabeth Fry visiting a prison.*
After a painting by Dighton.

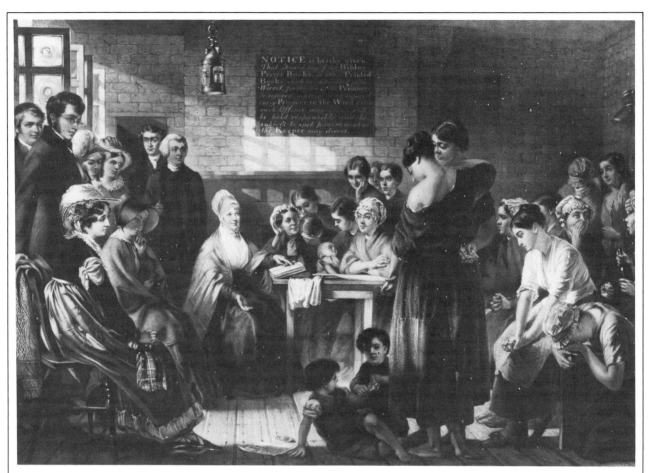

Elizabeth Fry preaching to women prisoners at Newgate in 1816. As well as interesting herself in prison reform, she also founded an order of nursing sisters. After a painting by Jerry Barrett.

When she was sixty, realizing that no training existed for the uneducated women who called themselves nurses, she drew up plans for a nurses' training home at a London hospital, 20 young women being selected for this purpose. At first these nurses were called Protestant Sisters of Charity, but they soon became known as Fry's Nurses. They wore a neat, plain uniform and received a stipend of £20 per annum, rising to £23 after three years' service, as compensation for their hard work and piety. At the home they were expected to attend prayers and were encouraged to read the Scriptures to their patients as well as to attend to their physical needs. They were the first trained nurses in England and, by the time the Crimean War broke out, there were 40 of these pious, respectable women with nursing experience. Some of them were to accompany Florence Nightingale to the Crimea.

In 1845, the Park Village Community, whose members were also known as Sisters of Mercy, was founded by the Rev. Edward Pusey's High Church movement. This was followed in 1848 by the Sellonite Sisters of Mercy and by St John's House, Westminster, another High Church sisterhood which sent six of its members with the Nightingale party.

The training of nurses

Most early attempts to train nurses had been undertaken by religious organizations. These, as has been seen, were Roman Catholic, and were strongly influenced by the French model. Apart from these there were a number of religious orders of men and women who devoted themselves to the service of the poor and afflicted. The first modern community, the Brothers of Charity, was founded in Belgium by Canon Triest in 1809. It subsequently established houses in England, Ireland and Canada. Similar organizations appeared in various parts of Europe and the United States, notably the Irish Sisters of Charity, started in 1815 by Mary Aikenhead. Another was the Sisters of Mercy founded by Catherine McAuley. Originally intended to provide a home for destitute girls, in 1830 it changed direction and concentrated on nursing. The Bermondsey branch, opened in 1839, was to supply five very able nuns for Florence Nightingale's party.

Much later, in 1859, a brilliant young woman, the Comtesse Agénor de Gasperin, who had original ideas and theories on the education and training of nurses, founded La

Source, the famous Swiss institution. The Comtesse felt that it was of the utmost importance that individuals should have their personal liberty, and that nurses should be salaried and not bound by vows. She backed up her ideas by buying the property in which the foundation had worked for many years and by providing it with a large sum of money, thus creating the first endowed training school.

Another inspired reformer who was to determine certain aspects of the future of nursing was Theodor Fliedner, the Lutheran pastor of the town of Kaiserswerth on the Rhine.

Fliedner was particularly interested in helping the families of prisoners, who suffered great deprivation while the bread-winner was incarcerated. An admirer of Elizabeth Fry, he met her in England during his travels. She was, in fact, the inspiration behind the scheme he carried out on returning to Kaiserswerth. It took him and his wife, Frederike, two years to found and staff an institution for training Protestant deaconesses to tend the sick. 'Of all my contemporaries,' wrote the pastor of Mrs Fry, 'none has exercised a like influence on my heart and life.'

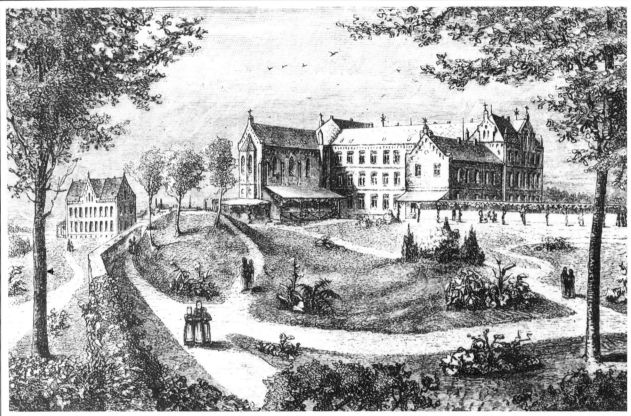

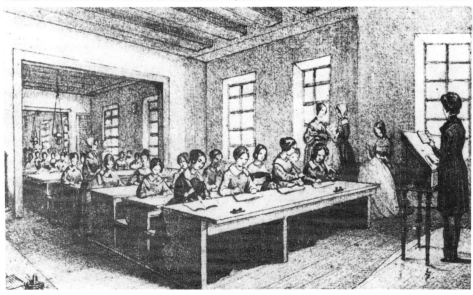

Above *A view of Kaiserswerth showing a women's hospital, one of several institutions, including orphanages and schools, opened by Theodor Fliedner in the 1830s and 1840s.*
Left *Deaconesses in class at Kaiserswerth c. 1840, undergoing the training which was to enable them to nurse the sick in hospitals. From a contemporary print.*

On 8 May 1840, Elizabeth Fry came to Kaiserswerth to find that her long-cherished dream of women leading useful lives had been realized. At the Institute she spoke to the 12 young women who were training to be teachers, while 20 deaconesses worked in the wards, nursing the sick.

Frederike Fliedner became the Institute's first superintendent. The experiment was an undoubted success, and soon Kaiserswerth could boast of a lunatic asylum, an orphanage, two schools and a hospital in which the deaconesses received their training. The work of the Fliedners was universally acclaimed and, when the pastor died in 1864, there were 32 deaconess houses (with 1600 deaconesses) scattered throughout Germany, Asia Minor and the United States.

Florence Nightingale

While the 18-year-old Victoria was learning to be queen, Florence Nightingale was still trying to find a purpose in life. Just before her 17th birthday she received what she believed to be a direct call from God. On 7 Feb. 1837, at her home at Embley, she wrote: 'God spoke and called me to His service.' What that service was to be she did not discover for 16 futile, desperate years. But during all that time her resolution to serve God did not falter and, in spite of continued opposition from her family, she began quietly equipping herself for the role she was to play in later life. In view of her talent for manipulation, her egotism and her steel will, it is surprising that she allowed herself to be dominated for so long by the wishes of a selfish mother, an hysterically jealous and possessive sister, and a peace-loving, weak dilettante of a father.

Despite the seemingly ideal life she led with her parents and her sister, Florence Nightingale did not have a happy childhood. She was obsessed with the idea that she was not like other people, that she was in fact a monster. She wrote that already at the age of six the life of ease and luxury she led was repugnant to her and began, like many imaginative children, to drift into a world of daydreams, into a kind of trance-like state which was an effective screen between herself and the real world.

Much is known of her struggles and inward feelings because of the avalanche of 'private notes' she wrote. Since she was too shy to confide her innermost thoughts to her immediate family, she scribbled them down on any bit of paper that came to hand. Naturally, her parents had no inkling of her secret life, or of her burning desire and determination to leave them in order to nurse the sick.

In 1842 she wrote in one of her private scribblings:

> 'My mind is absorbed with the idea of the
> sufferings of man, it besets me behind and before
> . . . all that poets sing of the glories of this world
> seem to me to be untrue. All the people I see are
> eaten up with care, poverty or disease.'

In 1842, in the midst of a social whirl, Florence called on her friends, the Baron and Baroness Bunsen. In a private talk with the Baron she asked his advice as to how she could help the sick and the suffering. He mentioned the work of Pastor Fliedner and his wife, at Kaiserswerth. At that time she had not thought of making nursing her vocation, but the idea of visiting the Fliedner's Institute entered her subconscious, where it was to lie dormant for some time.

Conditions in English hospitals

By 1845 the knowledge that her future lay in nursing the sick in hospitals had crystallized, and she began making a simple plan which she hoped would help her to overcome the difficulties she knew her family would put in her way. She realized that to become a nurse she would have to have training, and her idea was to persuade her parents to allow her to go for three months to Salisbury Infirmary to learn nursing. Salisbury was only a few miles from her home, the infirmary was well known and well run, and the head physician, Doctor Fowler, was an old friend.

Mrs Nightingale's reactions were predictable. She flew into a fury, accusing her daughter of having an attachment of which she was ashamed, with some 'low, vulgar surgeon'. In fact, there was some justification for Mrs Nightingale's horror at the thought of her gently nurtured daughter working in a hospital. In 1845 hospitals were grim places indeed. Fifteen years later, in her *Notes on Hospitals*, Florence Nightingale wrote:

> 'The floors were made of ordinary wood, which
> owing to lack of cleaning and sanitary
> conveniences for the patients' use, had become
> saturated with organic matter, which when washed
> gave off the smell of something quite other than
> soap and water. . . . The big bare wards were
> heated by minuscule fires at the end of each room,
> and in winter, windows were kept closed for
> warmth, sometimes for the whole of the winter.'

Nor were the patients who filled the hospitals in which Florence proposed nursing likely to lull the fears of her mother and sister. They came in diseased and dirty, and dirty they remained. She wrote:

> 'The nurses did not as a general rule wash patients,
> they could *never* wash their feet – and it was with
> difficulty and only in great haste that they could
> have a drop of water, just to *dab* their hands and
> face. The beds on which the patients lay were
> dirty. It was common practice to put a patient into
> the same sheets used by the last occupant of the
> bed, and mattresses were generally of flock,
> sodden, and seldom, if ever, cleaned.'

Florence Nightingale knew, however, that the real reason

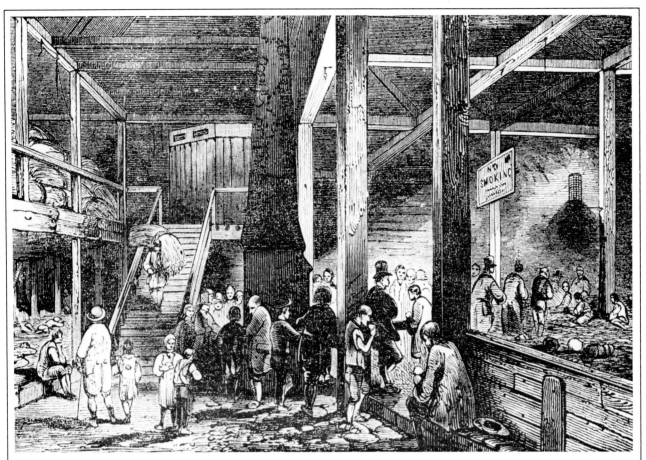

The male ward in a workhouse in the early 1840s. Conditions in such places were even worse than in hospitals and Florence Nightingale was in later years to help improve the status of workhouse infirmaries.

for her mother's anger at her wanting to nurse was conditioned by what she had been told about the notorious immorality of the women who nursed in the hospitals. 'It was preferred,' wrote Florence, 'that the nurses should be women who had lost their characters, i.e. should have one child.'

It is more than probable that both Florence Nightingale and her mother had read *Martin Chuzzlewit*, which Charles Dickens had written in 1844, and which contained two unfavourable descriptions of hired nurses. Many years later Dickens was to say that these portraits were not meant to be caricatures but were 'a fair representation of the hired attendant of the poor in sickness', Mrs Prig being 'a fair specimen of a hospital nurse'.

Mrs Nightingale's objections would have been further strengthened had she known that it was usual for the nurses to sleep in the wards they nursed, and fairly common for the nurses of male wards to sleep in the wards with the men.

In a letter written on 29 May 1894, Florence Nightingale described at length the sleeping quarters provided for the nursing staff in one of London's best-known hospitals:

'The nurses . . . slept in wooden cages on the
landing places outside the doors of the wards
where it was impossible for any woman of

character to sleep, where it was impossible for the
Night Nurse taking her rest in the day to sleep at
all owing to the noise, where there was not light
or air.'

Drink was another problem. 'The nurses are all drunkards, sisters and all', said the physician of a London hospital in 1851.

Once Florence Nightingale's 'plan' for nursing at the Salisbury Infirmary had been vetoed, the disappointed young woman returned to her own 'cage', where she suffered overwhelming attacks of depression. Even so, she continued to gather knowledge against the day when she would be 'free'.

She studied Blue Books and hospital reports. In 1838 a committee of doctors presented their report on the conditions of the poor in East London to the Poor Law Commissioners. Two years later a select committee presented its first report on the health of towns, and in 1842 the first report on the 'Sanitary Condition of the Labouring Classes' was published.

Facts and figures fascinated Florence Nightingale. She wrote off for further information about hospitals in France and Germany. She filled notebook after notebook with facts

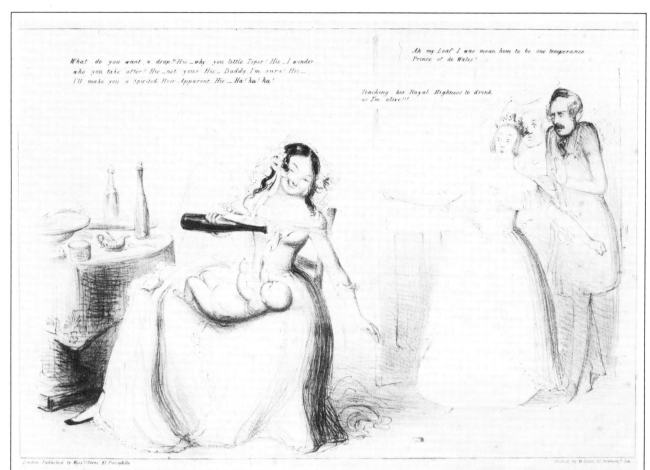

What do you want a drop? Hic — why you little Toper! Hic — I wonder who you take after? Hic — not your Hic — Daddy, I'm sure! Hic — I'll make you a Spirited Heir Apparent. Hic — Ha! ha! ha!

Ah my Loaf! I was mean him to be one temperance Prince of de Wales!

Teaching his Royal Highness to drink, as I'm alive!!!

ROYAL DRY NURSING EXTRAORDINARY.

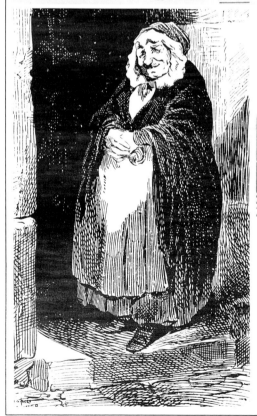

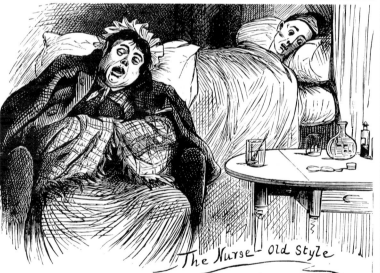

The Nurse — Old Style

Top *Apparently not even the highest in the land were safe from the attentions of the drunken nurse. Victoria and Albert discover the infant Prince of Wales being initiated into the pleasures of the bottle. Lithograph, c. 1842.*
Above *An intoxicated nurse dozes at the bedside of a patient. The quality of nursing improved dramatically in the course of the nineteenth century as this print of 1879 implies.*
Left *This portrait of a French nurse does not suggest that the profession as a whole enjoyed any greater public esteem on the other side of the Channel. Nineteenth-century engraving after Honoré Daumier.*

on sanitary conditions, a subject she steadily mastered and on which she would later become one of the foremost experts in the world.

The character of Florence Nightingale

The many saccharine biographies about Florence Nightingale failed to reveal her singularly complex character. She was a reformer who, in the words of F. B. Smith (*Florence Nightingale: Reputation and Power*, 1982), having discovered two great strengths in herself – 'an unyielding, unremitting drive to dominate her associates and opponents', and an extraordinarily perceptive understanding of the relations between individuals 'and the siting and working of things and of human beings' relations to them' – used these strengths as weapons to obtain what she wanted. Furthermore, though fragile and very feminine in appearance, she often thought of herself as a man. In one of her many conversations with her mother she tartly said, 'with my talents and my European reputation I am not going to stay dangling about my mother's drawing-room. I shall go out and look for work. . . . You must consider me married, or a son.'

Although many men fell in love with Florence Nightingale, and she was later to say that she had 'adored' the most favoured of her suitors, the rich, brilliant, amusing, and talented Richard Monkton Miles, she knew in her heart of hearts that she would never marry and must dedicate herself only to her life's work. All the same it took her seven long years before, in 1849, she finally gave Monkton Miles his dismissal. Her family were furious, and both he and she were broken-hearted, but she stood firm. She must wait for God to tell her what He wanted her to do.

Deeply shaken by her final parting with the man she loved, Florence was on the verge of a nervous breakdown. Her great friends, the Bracebridges, with whom she had already visited Rome, where she saw and studied the active Roman sisterhoods, were planning a trip to Egypt and Greece. They persuaded Mrs Nightingale to let Florence accompany them. However, the invalid still drooped, and did not revive until she was finally allowed by her parents to visit Kaiserswerth on the journey home.

Nursing at Kaiserswerth

She stayed there for two weeks, absorbing every detail of the work carried on by the Fliedners and their assistants. Yet, in spite of her admiration for the deaconesses, she had private reservations about certain aspects of the way in which the institute was run. 'The nursing was nil,' she wrote in 1897, 'the hygiene horrible. The hospital was certainly the worst part of Kaiserswerth. But never have I met with a higher

tone, a purer devotion than there. There was no neglect.' In 1860, when she founded her own nursing school, she copied some aspects of the Kaiserswerth administration, but organized it on totally different and more hygienic lines. The nursing, too, was of a much higher standard.

On her return from Germany Florence Nightingale went to her desk and, with amazing speed and concentration, wrote a 32-page pamphlet in less than a week. It told the 'unwanted women kept in busy idleness in England of work, happiness and comradeship waiting for them at Kaiserswerth.'

After her visit to Kaiserswerth, Florence was more determined than ever to take up nursing seriously. With the help of her friend, Doctor Manning, she went to Dublin, hoping to enter the hospital of the Sisters of Mercy who did magnificent work among the sick poor. Unfortunately for her the hospital was under repair and was being run by a depleted staff.

Undefeated, she again appealed to Doctor Manning and through him obtained a general permit to visit the establishments of L'Assistance Publique in Paris which, like the London County Council, was responsible for the administration of a number of hospitals, orphanages and other institutions in the French metropolis. Florence had also got permission to work at La Maison de Providence, the hospital of the Sisters of Charity in the Rue Oudinot. She was to train as a *postulante*, wear 'the dress of a nun', and 'render all necessary service to the sick' under the direction of the sisters, but she was to eat and sleep apart, and not enter the dormitory or the refectory of the sisters.

This plan too fell through because of the illness of her grandmother. During the time she nursed the old lady through her last days Florence mulled over yet another plan to escape.

Her friend, Liz Herbert, had let her know that the Institution for the Care of Sick Gentlewomen in Distressed Circumstances had got into deep trouble. It was to be moved from the premises it occupied and completely reorganized. Its managing committee was looking for a superintendent and Liz Herbert recommended Florence. She was interviewed and accepted for the post and, in spite of appalling scenes at home, she was immovable in her decision. On 12 Aug. 1853, free at last, she moved into the new premises at 1 Harley Street, London.

The committee, made up of wealthy and respectable gentlefolk, both male and female, was aghast when the new superintendent went into action. Her requirements were revolutionary. She insisted on hot water piped to every floor, and wanted a 'windlass' installation, a lift to bring up the patients' food. Brief though her visits had been to various hospitals and institutions, her razor-sharp mind and powers of observation had noted the many ways in which the logistics of nursing could be improved. She was an administrative genius, and she meant to get her own way. A dazed committee, impressed by their new superintendent's astonishing performance, let her have her head.

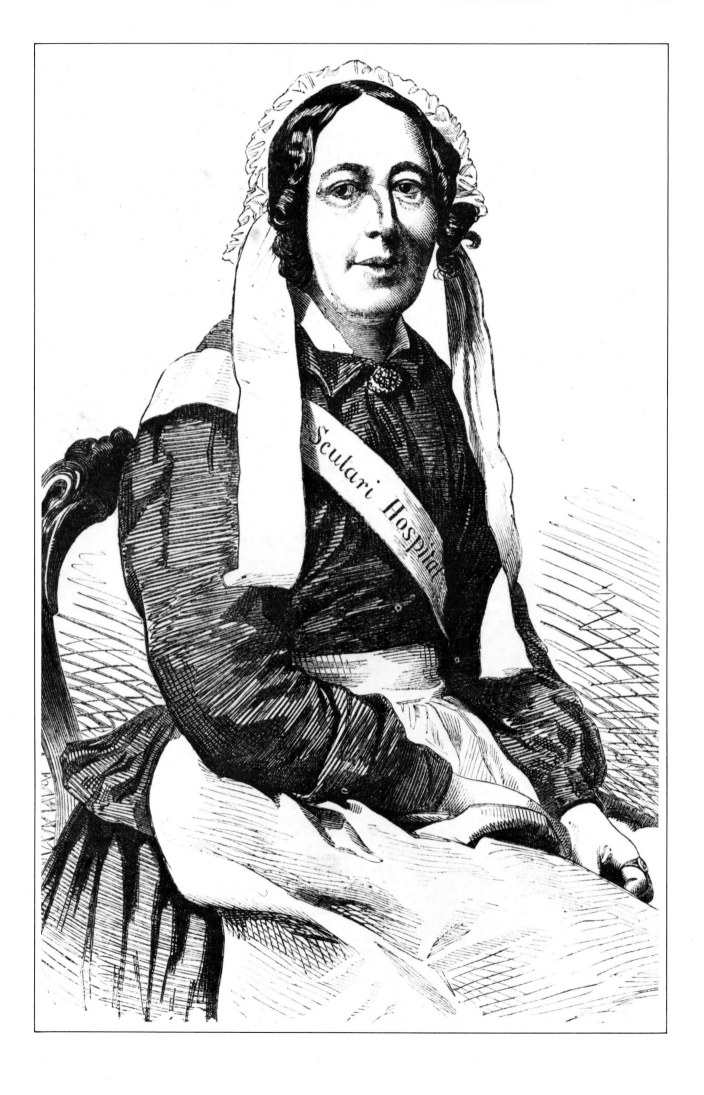

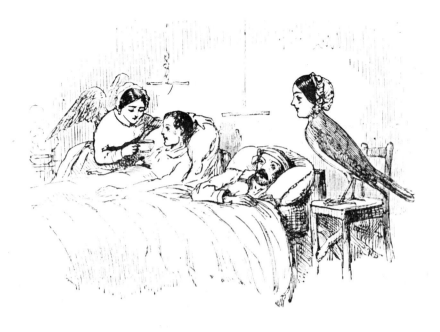

Military nursing and the Crimean War

Medical care for soldiers

From the earliest days help of a kind had been provided for sick and wounded fighting men. Physicians served in the armies of Alexander the Great, and at the time of the first Roman emperors there was, with each legion of 5000 men, a *medicus vulnerum* ('doctor of wounds'). Civil aid to troops on active service was first made available during the Crusades. In the Middle Ages some of the monastic orders sent their members out into the battlefields to give first aid to the wounded and, in some cases, to bring them back to the monastery infirmaries.

In England medical assistance for soldiers existed well before the fifteenth century, but was intended mainly for senior officers. In the reign of Edward II provision was made for one 'chirurgeon', whose pay was 4d. per day for every 1900 wounded. There was only one medical officer to care for the whole of Edward III's forces besieging Calais in 1355. Doctors were held in little esteem by military commanders, and in Henry V's Military Code physicians ranked after shoemakers and tailors, but before washerwomen!

Although there were many good and dedicated surgeons

they were outnumbered by legions of charlatans and quacks who manoeuvred their way into the army where rich pickings were to be had. These people, according to the famous military surgeon, Thomas Gale:

> . . . 'Be no chirugions, but manquillers,
> murtherers, and robbers of the people. Such are
> some hosiers, tailors, fletchers, minstrels, souters,
> horseleeches, juglers, witches, sorcerers, bawds,
> and a rabble of that sect, which would by lawes be
> driven from so divine an art, the exercise of
> which, for want of knowledge, bringeth sometimes
> loss of member, sometimes of life, and sometimes
> both of limme and life.'

From the sixteenth century onwards, commanders began to show a more humanitarian regard for the sufferings of their troops and, during the seventeenth, eighteenth and early nineteenth centuries, nearly 300 treaties were drawn up relating to the exchange of prisoners of war and the care of the wounded and the sick.

Nursing the wounded

English soldiers were, in general, nursed by male orderlies, although, in some cases, wives and camp followers did assist the orderlies to look after the wounded. Nursing in war was, in the main, a haphazard affair, depending on the charity and good intentions of a number of humane and pious women. Queen Isabella of Spain (1451–1504) is said to have

Top *A contemporary illustration entitled 'Wounded Soldiers and Nightingales' showing how Florence Nightingale's work in the Crimea had caught the public imagination.*
Opposite *A Scutari Hospital nurse, one of the contingent chosen by Florence Nightingale to accompany her to the Crimea. Engraving from a photograph taken in Dec. 1855.*

been the first to introduce camp hospitals in the wars of her reign. These are described as 'large tents' (*tiendas grandes*) equipped with beds, where the sick were cared for by 'decent women specially engaged for this purpose'.

In England under the Commonwealth a courageous and caring woman called Elizabeth Alkin did her best in 1653 to help the wounded sailors who were landed in East Anglia after various naval engagements. She appears to have worked in Ipswich and Harwich, using her own money to provide for the men in her care. Equally dedicated to helping the wounded was Soeur Marthe (Anne Biget, 1749–1824) who, in the Napoleonic Wars, did all she could to help wounded French, Spanish and English prisoners.

But, generally speaking, the only women who nursed in an army were untrained camp followers. In 1777, at the time of the American War of Independence, George Washington ordered that 'a proportionate number of women, to the sick of each regiment, shall be sent to the hospitals at Mendham and Black River, to attend the sick as nurses.'

Martha Ross and Ann Winzer were two heroic women who nursed the wounded on the field of battle. Martha, who had followed her husband, found herself in the thick of the great battle fought at Fontenoy on 1 May 1745. Her assiduous care of the wounded and dying men was noticed by the commander-in-chief, William, Duke of Cumberland, who commended her for her 'intrepidity and assistance to the wounded.'

Ann Winzer is described on her tombstone as 'A Waterloo heroine who assisted at that great battle, A.D. 1815, by aiding and assisting the sick and wounded.' It is further recorded that the tombstone was set up 'as a tribute of respect to a long life spent in true and faithful service, by the kindness of Colonel Astell and many other officers.'

During the Peninsular War women ceased to be employed as nurses, but continued to officiate as cooks and washerwomen. By 1832 women were no longer employed in regimental hospitals in any capacity whatsoever.

Military hospitals

At the end of the seventeenth century, when staff hospitals first came into use, they were of two kinds: the fixed hospital, which developed into a general hospital, and the marching hospital, which was later to become the 'flying' hospital. The marching hospital was reasonably mobile, and had its own tentage and transport wagons. Its function was to act as a casualty clearing station between the regimental hospital and the fixed hospital. It was an essential part of the system, since it meant there were clear administrative and transport links between the front and the rearguard.

Flying hospitals were discarded during the Peninsular War because their transport wagons obstructed the roads. This move was to have grave repercussions later on, during the Crimean War, since the staff surgeon, acting as senior

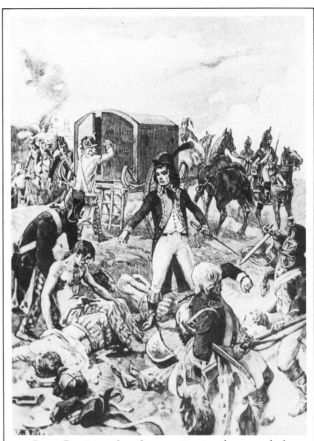

Baron Dominique Jean Larrey supervises the removal of wounded soldiers from the battlefield. A surgeon in the French army during the Napoleonic Wars, Larrey is credited with the introduction of the so-called 'flying ambulances' which were used to transport the wounded to hospital.

medical officer to the brigade, then had to apply to the commissary general for transport to evacuate his sick and wounded, which meant there was a great divide between the regiments at the front and the general hospital at Scutari.

In wartime general hospitals, as opposed to regimental hospitals, were accepted as a necessary evil, but in peacetime their numbers were severely reduced. For a long time no arrangements were made for the sick returning from duty overseas. The transport commissions were responsible for them as long as they were being transported, but what happened to them after they had reached their destination was nobody's concern, with the result that helpless sick and wounded soldiers were left to fend for themselves.

Their plight was slightly relieved in 1781 when the first general military hospital was opened in England. Between 1802 and 1806 the general hospitals at Gosport, Plymouth, and Deal were closed on grounds of economy when it was discovered that it cost 17d. a day to keep a man in a general hospital, and only 10d. a day in a regimental hospital.

After Waterloo the government made drastic economies and the Army Medical Department was cut to the bone. The net result was that when war was declared in the Crimea, no general hospital had been established for 40 years.

The Crimean War

In Sept. 1853 Turkey declared war on Russia. A combined French and English fleet was sent to the Black Sea, and war between Russia on the one hand and France and England on the other followed in March 1854. In June a British army landed at Varna, on the western shore of the Black Sea, to go to the assistance of the Turks, who were being besieged by the Russians. The Turks managed without their aid. However, cholera broke out among the British troops and a horrifying shambles ensued. The soldiers were re-embarked in a number of inadequate transports, leaving behind much of their medical equipment and supplies. They sailed across the Black Sea to the Crimean peninsula, with the object of capturing the naval base at Sebastopol. They disembarked at a bay called Kalamita, where they fought the savage and bloody battle of the Alma.

It was a victory paid for dearly by the men who took part in the fighting. The wounded survivors were almost worse off than their dead comrades, for they lay on the ground or on straw mixed with manure in a farmyard, dying like flies. There were no bandages, no splints, no chloroform and no morphia. The surgeons worked by moonlight because there were no candles or lamps. Over 1000 cholera cases were sent back to Scutari.

The hospital at Scutari

The British public, proud of their glorious fighting men, knew nothing of the horrors that awaited the sick and wounded when they were finally landed at Scutari. Here was the vast barracks which had been the headquarters of the Turkish artillery. These had been handed over to the British authorities who imagined that the barrack hospital, known as the General Hospital, would be large enough to house the terrible casualties. But the cholera epidemic produced total confusion. The hospital was already packed to overflowing with the cholera cases sent back after the landing at Kalamita. Supplies were totally insufficient and there were not enough doctors. Dr Menzies, the senior medical officer, was appalled at the magnitude of the task he and his staff had to cope with. While he was trying to sort out the hospital, he was told that many battle casualties from the Alma, as well as 1000 cholera cases, were on their way to the overcrowded General Hospital.

Dr Menzies gave orders that the artillery barracks should immediately be converted into a hospital in order to receive the new influx of sick and wounded. The enormous building was filthy, bare and falling to bits. There was no labour to clean it and no equipment to furnish it.

When the men finally arrived at the barrack hospital there

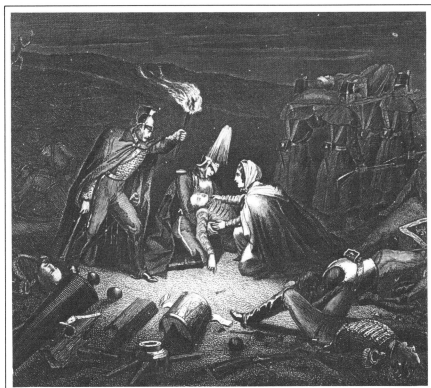

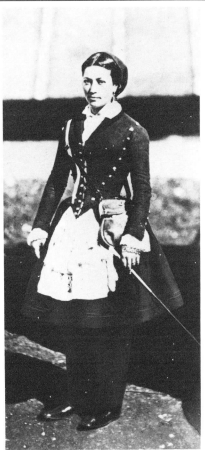

Above *A nurse tends a wounded soldier after the Battle of the Alma in the early stages of the Crimean War.*
Right *A French cantinière during the Crimean War who also gave assistance and first aid to wounded soldiers.*

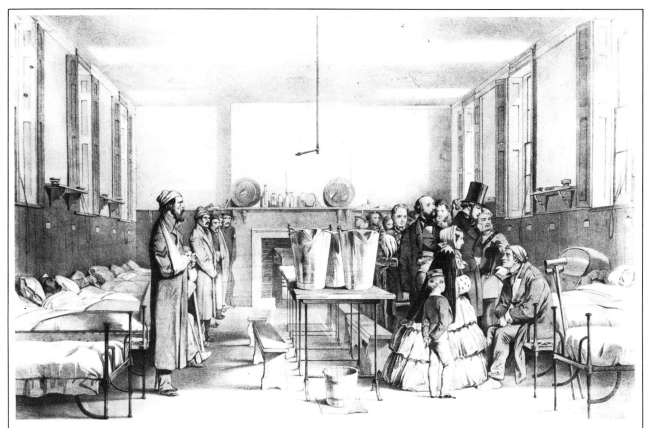

Queen Victoria and Prince Albert, with their children, visiting sick and wounded soldiers from the Crimean War at the Brompton Hospital, Chatham.

were no beds, so they lay rolled up in blankets sodden with blood and faeces. They had no food because there was no kitchen and no cooking facilities. Though they moaned for water, there were no buckets, cups or drinking utensils. There were no operating tables and few doctors.

Queen Victoria always felt most strongly that the army was her army, the soldiers her 'dear soldiers', and her pride in them was very real. Her horror, therefore, when she read what the war correspondent of *The Times*, W. H. Russell, had to say about conditions in the Crimea, was transmitted in a series of seismic shock waves from her to the prime minister and downwards. Russell did not mince words. He stated on 12 Oct. that the military hospitals had not got 'the commonest appliances of a workhouse sick ward', and that 'the men must die through the medical staffs of the British Army having forgotten that old rags were necessary for the dressing of wounds.'

Florence Nightingale to the rescue

Russell's reports from the front aroused not only the indignation of the queen, but that of many of her subjects. 'Why,' asked one reader, in a passion, 'have we no Sisters of Charity?' At that time no women nurses were regularly employed in British army hospitals, but in France the soldiers were nursed by the Sisters of Charity. *The Illustrated London News* caught on to the idea and published a picture of the good nuns at work in a ward of their hospital.

Florence Nightingale wrote offering her services to her friend, Liz Herbert, wife of Sidney Herbert, then by chance holding the office (now obsolete) of Secretary at War. By the strangest of coincidences, Herbert had written to Florence requesting her to go to the Crimea, taking with her a group of nurses to work in the military hospitals. Their letters crossed in the post.

In his letter Herbert formally asked Florence Nightingale to take charge of an official scheme for introducing female nurses into the hospitals of the British army. This was indeed a bold move, and one fraught with difficulties. It was an innovation which would shock many people but, although neither he nor Florence Nightingale realized it, his decision opened up a new profession to Englishwomen of good birth and gave immediate status to nursing.

When it was discovered that various religious bodies had already arranged to send out parties of nurses to Scutari, Florence Nightingale made it plain that there was to be only one leader, only one administrator, and that was herself. As always, she got her way, and took into her 'official' party those nurses chosen by her selection committee, composed of her friends Mrs Herbert, Lady Canning and Mrs Brace-

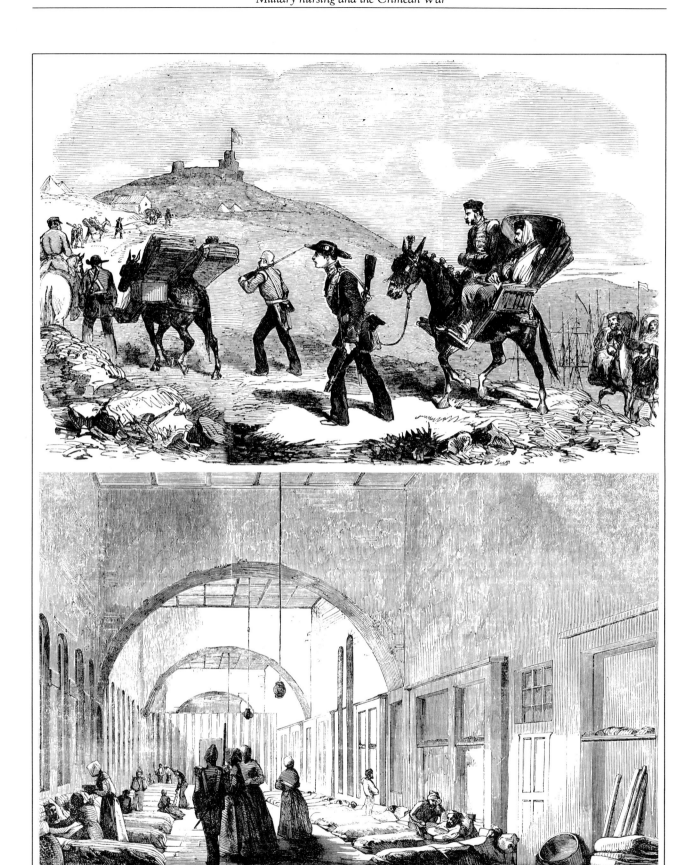

Top *Wounded soldiers being transported to hospital by mule. Illustrated London News, 1855.*
Above *The Barrack Hospital at Scutari which was to be the scene of so much unnecessary suffering among sick and wounded British soldiers before the arrival of Florence Nightingale. Illustrated London News, 1854.*

bridge. Florence Nightingale herself was busy consolidating her authority with governments and heads of religious houses.

The contingent of nurses finally brought together comprised ten Roman Catholic sisters from Bermondsey and Norwood, eight Anglican sisters from an order called Sisters of Mercy, founded at Davenport a few years previously, six nurses from St John's House and fourteen lay nurses from different hospitals, plus Mrs Clarke, Florence Nightingale's housekeeper from Upper Harley Street. Also travelling in the party were Mr and Mrs Bracebridge who, being close friends, could be counted on for moral support.

Florence Nightingale had decided that her nurses must wear uniforms. These were ordered in a rush and, apart from being badly designed and cut, they were extremely unattractive, consisting of an ill-fitting grey tweed dress, a grey worsted jacket, a short woollen cloak, and a white cap. A holland scarf, embroidered with the words 'Scutari Hospital' in red thread, was worn around the shoulders. Only the nuns and sisters in the party were allowed to wear their own habits or uniform.

Though morale was high when the party left on 21 Oct. 1854, it sank to zero during the eight days of their journey while the ill-found tub, the *Vectis*, bucketed its way through the heavy storms which went on unabated throughout the voyage. Florence Nightingale suffered from violent sea sickness, as did most members of her party.

Their arrival was as cheerless as the voyage. It was pouring with rain, and the steep slopes to the barrack hospital were a sea of mud littered with refuse. Tired, cold and exhausted from the sea-voyage, the nurses, clutching their belongings, climbed the slope and, spattered with mud, entered the hospital.

With a sinking heart Florence Nightingale viewed her surroundings. The vast building was a shambles and, as she was soon to discover, the methods by which hospitals were supplied were so compartmentalized, so tied up with red tape that by the time rations were actually distributed to the men they might well suffer chronic indigestion caused by the badly cooked lumps of meat given them. Food intended for invalids, such as sago, rice, arrowroot and port wine, was ordered through so many channels and passed through so many departments that the 'invalids' were either dead or had completely recovered by the time these comforts reached them.

As Florence Nightingale was soon to discover, the hospital was short of even the most elementary eating utensils, such as forks, knives and plates. Officials were trained to penny-pinch and to avoid responsibility. No orders given by a woman were going to make them change their habits. The doctors, too, made life difficult for Florence Nightingale and her nurses. They were furious that these women should have been sent out to 'hamper' them in their work.

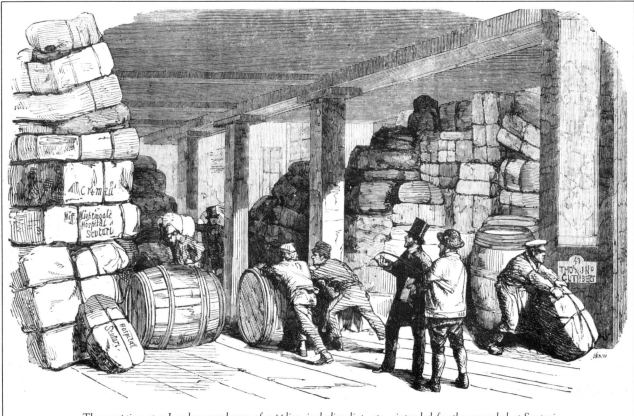

The reception at a London warehouse of supplies, including lint, etc., intended for the wounded at Scutari.

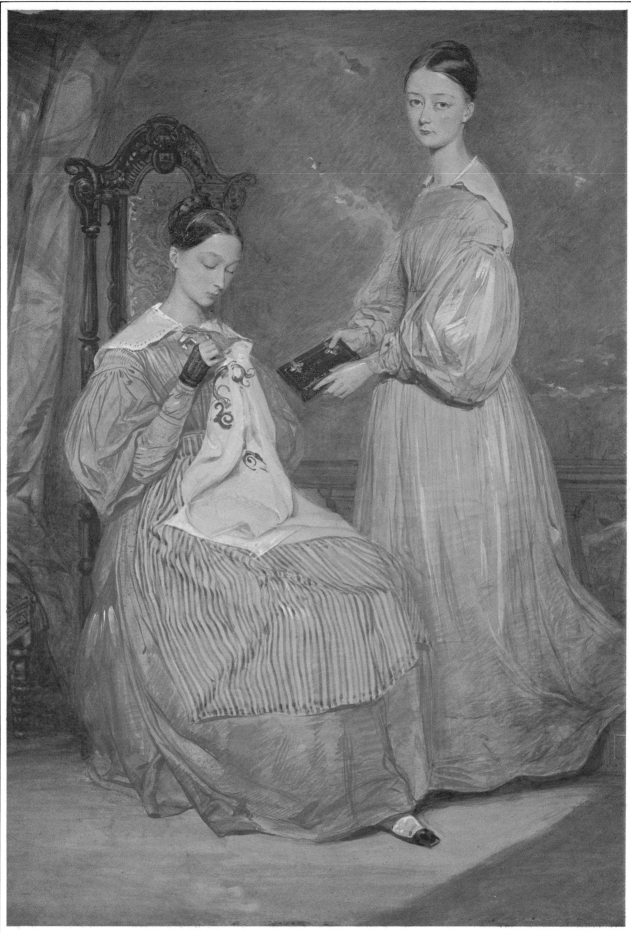

Above *Florence Nightingale (seated) with her sister, Frances Parthenope, afterwards Lady Verney. Despite the appearance of domestic tranquillity, Florence's relationship with her jealous and possessive sister was never a very easy one. Watercolour by William White, c.1836.*

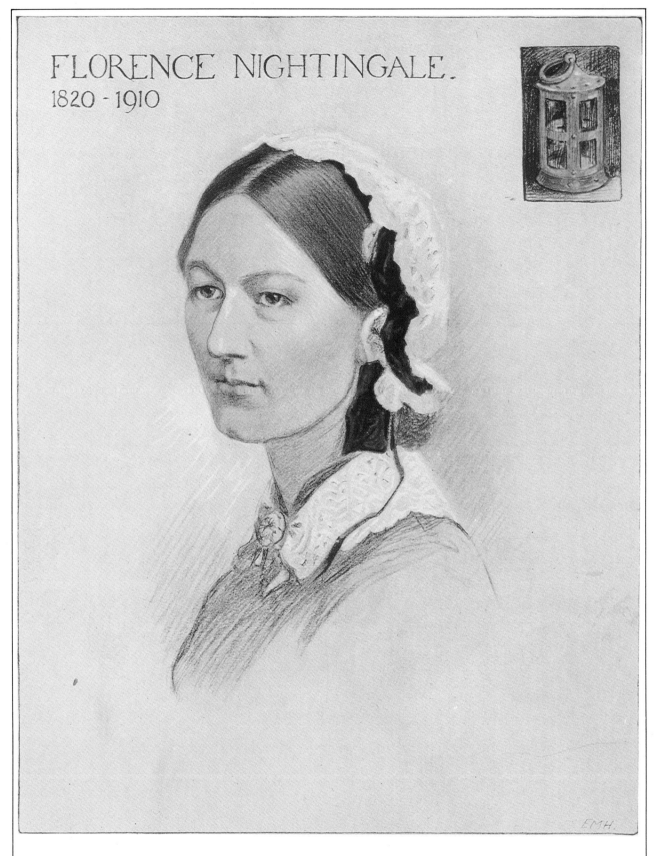

FLORENCE NIGHTINGALE.
1820 - 1910

Portrait of Florence Nightingale. Her conviction that her decision to become a nurse was divinely inspired enabled her to overcome the many obstacles placed in her path. She was the first woman to be awarded the Order of Merit (1907).

Florence Nightingale's achievement

Florence Nightingale ignored all the obstacles put in her way. She said nothing when shown her quarters and those of her nurses. They had been allotted six rooms, one of which was a kitchen, and another a closet, ten feet square, was supposed to house 40 persons. The rooms were damp, dirty and unfurnished. There were no means of cooking and no beds save Turkish divans, raised wooden platforms on which bedding was placed. Only there was no bedding. There was a shortage of water, and of lamps and candles.

The Lady Superintendent now showed her mettle. The first task was to clean the place. Three hundred scrubbing brushes were urgently requisitioned, and the wards freed of bugs and filth. From her own stores she provided bedding, medicine, clothing and 'comforts'. As soon as the situation had become clear, in England *The Times* had set up a fund to help with the buying of necessities. Under the direction of the surgeons, Florence Nightingale's nurses took up their duties which consisted of preparing invalid meals, making beef tea, making up palliasses, writing letters for the illiterate, and providing fresh clothing and bedding.

The real nursing, dressing of wounds and washing of patients was still carried out by the male orderlies. 'The nuns' and ladies' refined feelings, reinforced by the men's modesty, generally inhibited them from dealing with the men's evacuations, and with wounds to their abdominal regions.'

In the face of opposition, not only from doctors, administrators and meddlers such as the wife of the British ambassador, Lady Stratford, Florence Nightingale also had to contend with personality clashes among her nurses. Many of the lay nurses behaved badly. They got drunk, allowed the patients too much latitude, and ceaselessly criticized the nuns and the Lady Superintendent. By Christmas 1854 she had dismissed some 13 of her original party, leaving her with 25 nuns and nurses to look after 11,000 men suffering from scurvy, dysentery, exposure and starvation diseases. Very few had war wounds. She continued to work steadily through the day and half the night. Gradually she managed to establish some sort of order out of the chaos and, when it became known that she had a large sum of money – over £30,000 – collected from various sources and to be used entirely at her discretion, it was to the Lady Superintendent that requests were made for all the extras and comforts.

From the start Florence Nightingale made it clear that she expected to be obeyed and that cleanliness, air, light and warmth were to be her main weapons in combating the horrors of the barrack hospital. She was not only an administrative genius but also a very practical and efficient woman, and by the end of Dec. 1854 she had, to all intents and purposes, become purveyor to the hospital, supplying, on the requisition of the medical officers, some 6000 shirts, 2000 socks, and 500 pairs of drawers. With money one could obtain anything, and Constantinople was one of the great market places of the world.

Alexis Soyer

Florence Nightingale's fight for better food for her patients found a new champion and ally in Alexis Soyer, former chef of the Reform Club, and one of the greatest creative cooks of all time. Soyer was also the inventor of a number of remarkable and useful gadgets for the kitchen. But of all his inventions the most notable was his portable cooking stove, suitable for use in camps or hospitals, which consumed a minimum of fuel. Soyer had a model made up in a few days, and took it to the War Office where it was enthusiastically received. When it was manufactured, Brunel, the great engineer, decided to make use of it at the base hospitals at Smyrna and Rankoi. The stove was eventually adopted for use by the entire army and, as late as 1935, was 'among the most essential articles of camp equipment'.

Appalled by what he had read about the state of the field kitchens and the lack of cooking facilities in the hospitals in the Crimea, Soyer, who had many friends in high places, persuaded the British government to send him out to improve the food and the insanitary conditions in the field and hospital kitchens.

Soyer fought bureaucracy as fiercely and successfully as did Florence Nightingale. It was she who outlined to him the system by which patients in a military hospital were fed. A particular patient was placed on full, half, low or spoon diet. The daily allowance for full diet was one pound of meat, one pound of bread, one pound of potatoes, two pints of tea, and half a pint of porter. Half diet was exactly one half of this diet, low diet one half again of that, and spoon diet was simply one pound of bread and one pint of tea. Extras might be given only to men on spoon diet.

Apart from the endless administrative red tape which required chits to be signed and countersigned by surgeons, assistant surgeons, medical officers and so on down the line, Soyer discovered the the only apparatus left for cooking by the Turks when they vacated the barrack hospital consisted of 13 large copper boilers in a kitchen of sorts at the end of the yard.

Meat was issued to the ward orderlies by a single official. Many of the orderlies did not get their joints and take them to the kitchens until well into the afternoon. They had, as Soyer noted, '. . . most curious methods of marking their different lots. Some used a piece of red cloth cut from an old jacket; others half a dozen buttons tied together; old knives, forks, scissors. One in particular had hit upon the idea of tying a pair of snuffers to the lot. All this rubbish was daily boiled with the meat. Each orderly then took his bundle of joints to his own bed, where he divided the meat into portions and distributed the rations to his patients. . . .' When the food did come, it was often uneatable, being either parboiled or raw. 'The waste in the wards,' said Florence Nightingale, 'was enormous because the men were unable to eat diets so badly cooked.'

Soyer, having discovered that the men lived mainly on a

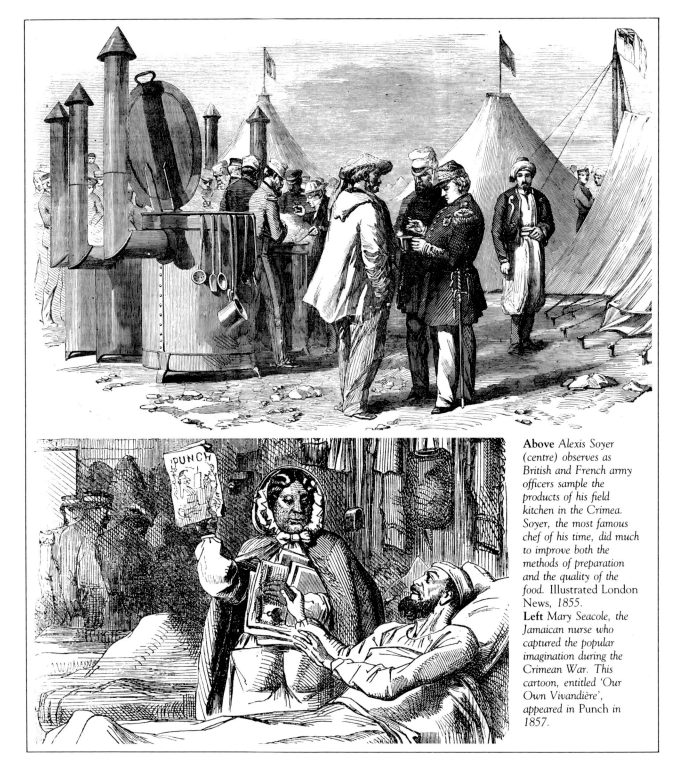

Above *Alexis Soyer (centre) observes as British and French army officers sample the products of his field kitchen in the Crimea. Soyer, the most famous chef of his time, did much to improve both the methods of preparation and the quality of the food.* Illustrated London News, *1855.*
Left *Mary Seacole, the Jamaican nurse who captured the popular imagination during the Crimean War. This cartoon, entitled 'Our Own Vivandière', appeared in* Punch *in 1857.*

regimen of biscuits, salt pork and rum, began at once to experiment and improvise. Almost immediately he contrived new dishes from standard rations, and invented a kind of ground-baked peas-meal which, with the addition of boiling water, became a thick comforting soup made quickly in an emergency.

Another colourful figure of the Crimean War was Mary Seacole who, according to the engraving on the headstone of her tomb in Shepherd's Bush, 'was a notable nurse who cared for the sick and wounded in the West Indies, Panama, and on the battlefields of the Crimea 1854–1856'. This extraordinary woman from Jamaica had many adventures before she finally arrived in the Crimea. She had an interview with Florence Nightingale, no mean feat when one considers that virtually every instant of the life of the Lady Superintendent was taken up with her work, and was absolutely enchanted with the slim young woman of whom she was to write in a rather dramatic fashion:

'Florence Nightingale, that Englishwoman whose name shall never die, but sound like music on the lips of British men until the hour of doom.'

Strangely enough, while Florence Nightingale's patients were practically starving, Mrs Seacole's storerooms in 'The British Hotel', an establishment which offered to vary the diet of the British officers, were stuffed with a vast selection of 'preserved provisions, salmon, lobsters and oysters', also in tins, which, with onions, butter, eggs and salt were very good. She had also managed to get quantities of game, wild fowl, vegetables (also preserved), sardines, and currant jelly. Anyone dropping in at her hotel was almost sure to find 'a good joint of mutton, a curry, an Irish stew or some capital meat pies'.

Whenever possible, Mother Seacole, as she was known, packed large bags with provisions, together with her 'medical equipment', lint, bandages, needle and thread and, having loaded these on to two mules, made her way to the scene of action where she was often under fire.

The Lady with the Lamp

Six months after the arrival of Florence Nightingale there was a marked improvement in the condition of the hospital at Scutari, and she felt she should go to the Crimea and visit the hospitals to which she had sent some of her nurses. After a very uncomfortable crossing she and her party arrived at Balaclava on 8 May 1855. What the Lady Superintendent had suffered in the way of hardships at Scutari was as nothing compared to the frightful conditions she now encountered. The peninsula was mountainous, distances between the hospitals were great and roads were non-existent. Undeterred, she went on horseback to visit the sick, or was transported in a small carriage, which had a hood to protect her from the elements.

Besides Soyer and a French chef, the party included Soyer's secretary, a 'gentleman of colour', Mr Bracebridge, and a boy of 12, named Robert Robinson, a drummer invalided out of the 68th Light Infantry. He described himself as 'Miss Nightingale's man', saying that he had 'forsaken his instruments in order to devote his civil and military career to Miss Nightingale'. He carried her letters and messages, escorted her to and from hospitals, and was in charge of the famous lamp. He was, said Soyer, who teased him about his age, 'a regular enfant de troupe, full of wit and glee':

Tired and weakened by the great efforts she had made, Florence Nightingale now fell victim to the malady known as 'Crimean Fever', but which may well have been a virulent attack of typhus. As soon as she was convalescent, pale, emaciated, and very frail, the woman whom the soldiers had christened 'The Lady with the Lamp' pressed on with her duties. The news of her illness and recovery had spread

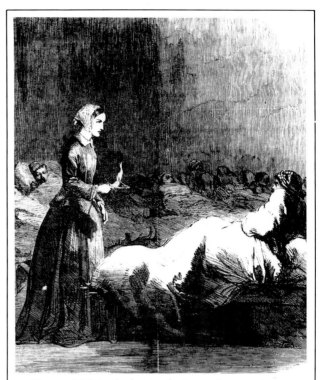

Florence Nightingale, bearing the famous lamp, makes her way round the wards at Scutari. Although she was not always popular with the military authorities, the common soldiers regarded her with the greatest esteem and affection.
Illustrated London News, 1855.

throughout England, where the reports of her activities at Scutari had made her the heroine of the hour.

One of the nurses described accompanying her on her night vigils:

' . . . It seemed an endless walk. . . . As we passed the silence was profound; very seldom did a moan or cry from those deeply suffering fall on our ears. A dim light burned here and there. Miss Nightingale carried her lantern which she would set down before she bent over the patients.'

The troops worshipped her. A soldier wrote:

'What a comfort it was to see her pass even. She would speak to one, and nod and smile to many more; but she could not do it to all you know. We lay there by hundreds; but we could kiss her shadow as it fell, and lay our heads on the pillow again content.'

At the end of Feb. 1855 the Secretary for War, Lord Panmure, sent out a sanitary commission to investigate the state of the buildings used as hospitals and of the camps both at Scutari and in the Crimea. Though Florence Nightingale's name did not appear, it was obvious that she was the driving force behind the investigation. 'This Commission,' she said later, 'saved the British Army.'

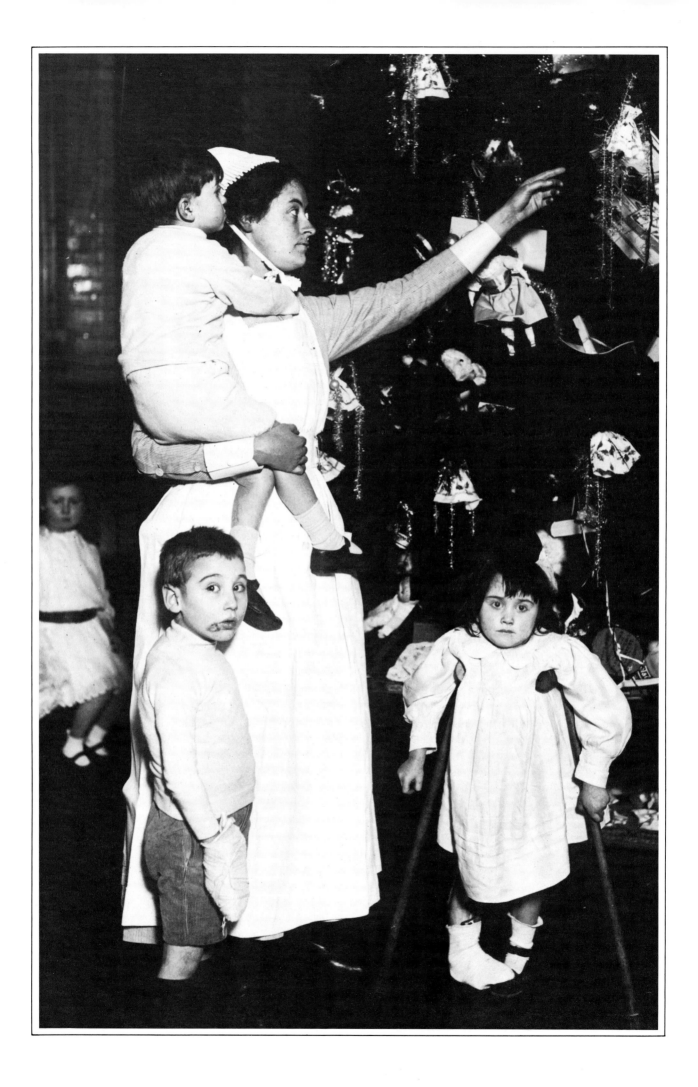

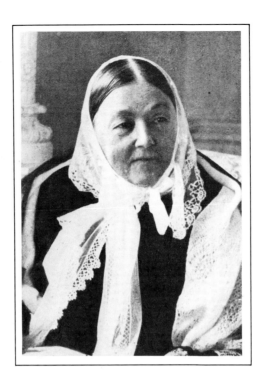

Modern nursing comes into being

The Nightingale Training School

Florence Nightingale returned from the Crimea in a blaze of glory. Aged 36, she was an international heroine. She had the support and admiration of her sovereign, underlined by the gift of a large, ornate brooch designed by Prince Albert, and was the first woman to be thus decorated for public services. She was also completely her own mistress and would never again allow her life to be ruled by her family.

Though physically weakened by her illness and the conditions under which she had worked in the Crimea, Florence Nightingale was determined to change the appalling treatment of 'her' sick and invalided soldiers by reforming the general standards of health of the British army. This news was not received with any enthusiasm by the War Office, who had hoped that this powerful and influential woman would, in peacetime, return to her own field of hospital management.

Meanwhile a committee had been formed to 'give expression to a general feeling that the services of Miss Nightingale in the Hospitals of the East demanded the grateful recognition of the British people.' So much money came in that it was decided to set up a Nightingale Fund to enable her 'to establish and control an institute for the training, sustenance and protection of nurses, paid and unpaid'.

Florence Nightingale was grateful, but showed no great eagerness to make use of the £40,000 at her disposal. She was occupied with her work for the royal commissions which she did not finish until 1859. Only then did she turn her attention to the founding of the Nightingale Training School. Naturally it was expected that she would head whatever school or institution she founded, but she had no intention of nursing again or of taking charge of any nursing establishment. She much preferred to pull strings behind the scenes to further her great projects of reform.

The whole idea of a training school for nurses was looked on with great disfavour by many influential doctors. J. F. South, consulting surgeon at St Thomas' Hospital, made it clear that so far as he and many of his colleagues were concerned, the nursing establishments in the leading hospitals were excellent, and he could not see 'that they are likely to be improved by any special institution for training'. Nurses learn by experience, he argued, and needed only the simplest instructions for making up things like poultices.

Florence Nightingale paid not the slightest attention to the warnings of the doctors that training schools for nurses would endanger the patients by giving the nurses too much control. She carefully worked out the structure of her school and then consulted a number of able women with expertise and experience in all aspects of nursing and hospital management, both in England and abroad.

Having assimilated all available information she and her advisers looked round for a suitable London hospital to house their training school. Their choice fell on St Thomas',

Top A photograph of Florence Nightingale in 1891. A semi-invalid for much of her long life, she nevertheless continued to take an active interest in all aspects of nursing reform and health education.
Opposite A Christmas party at the Hospital for Sick Children, Great Ormond Street, London, in 1919. Established in 1851, it was the country's first children's hospital.

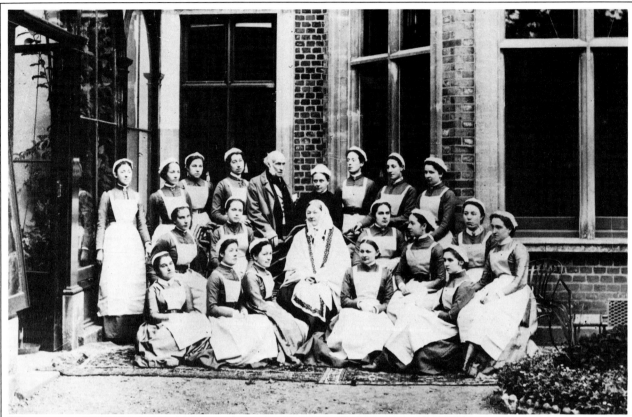

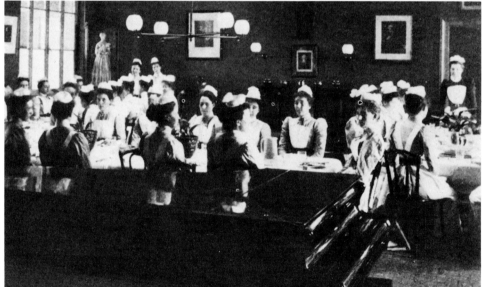

Above *Florence Nightingale seated at the centre of a group of nurses from London hospitals at Claydon House in 1886. Her brother-in-law, Sir Harry Verney, is standing behind her.*

Left *A dining room in the Nightingale Home and Training School for Nurses at St Thomas' Hospital in the early twentieth century. Its founder took a keen interest in its development over the years and made strenuous efforts to ensure the maintenance of high standards.*

mainly one suspects, because of Florence Nightingale's admiration for its matron, Mrs Wardroper. This refined, well-bred, efficient, and well-educated widow, with four children, was the prototype of what Florence Nightingale felt the matron of a large hospital should be. Mrs Wardroper was a lady and had authority, and was respected by doctors and staff alike. Furthermore, she could be expected to carry out to the letter the precepts laid down in Florence Nightingale's excellent book, *Notes on Nursing*, which was published in 1859.

Although almost entirely dealing with home nursing, the book is full of sound common sense as to the treatment and welfare of patients in any environment. It advocated the use of fresh air, quiet, a wholesome but pleasant diet well served, and the provision of fresh flowers and plants. Nurses should be gentle and reassuring. Their particular training, said the writer, would give them a better understanding of the needs of those under their care.

Florence Nightingale gave secular vocational nursing an important new meaning in Victorian Britain. It became identified in the public mind with sanctified duty, and parents now felt that in allowing their daughters to follow her example they were doing a service to their country. Many young women with no prospects other than those of being governesses or companions to exigent old ladies would have cause to be grateful to the Lady with the Lamp.

The late age of marriage, low marriage rates, wars and migration had created a pool of spinster labour. The single woman was prevented by powerful social pressures from competing in almost any field against the dominant male sex. If she did not marry, she must either remain at home to do the flowers, help her mother arrange tea-parties, or carry broth and jelly to the sick poor. Until the Nightingale Training School opened, a young lady of good family would never have been allowed to mix with the 'Sairey Gamps', whom their parents thought of as typical nurses.

Yet another cogent reason for Florence Nightingale's choice of St Thomas' Hospital as a suitable venue for her training school was the fact that she had been privately advised that the ancient hospital was going to be moved from Southwark, where it had been since the twelfth century, and was to be completely rebuilt. As she had her own views on the construction of hospitals and on accommodation for nursing staff, she wanted the new St Thomas' to be built on the 'pavilion' plan which she felt was eminently practical.

Her next move was to conclude business arrangements with the governors of the hospital, who were to have no voice in the selection of the Nightingale trainees. She had made it plain that she wanted probationers, and not novices with their overtones of religious orders. At the beginning it was thought that 'the candidates who are best qualified for the ordinary duties of the hospital nurse appear to be daughters of small farmers who have been used to household work – and well-educated domestic servants.' Stress was laid on high moral character, and in fact the first probationer to enrol at the Nightingale Training School was only permitted to do so by her mother on condition that she was never allowed to enter a male ward.

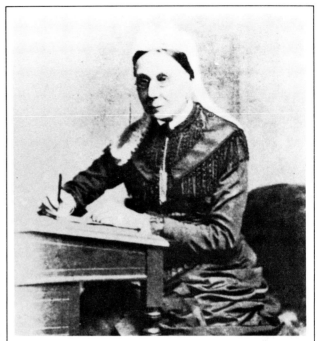

Mrs Wardroper, who became matron of St Thomas' Hospital in 1854, was in the opinion of Florence Nightingale admirably suited to take charge of the training of probationer nurses under the Nightingale system, which began at St Thomas' in July 1860.

Lady-pupils

In May 1860 advertisements appeared seeking young ladies for nursing training. The response was not overwhelming and it became obvious that recruitment was not going to be easy. However, on 9 July 1860, 15 hand-picked probationers entered the Nightingale Training School and the pattern for modern nursing came into being.

Florence Nightingale had dictated the rules from her sickbed. All trainee nurses were to live in at the hospital, and each probationer was to record in a daily ward book her duties and observations of patients, which were to be sent monthly to Florence Nightingale. These ward books, together with the entries in the discipline register, were to be reviewed before any certificate was issued by the Fund Committee, then consisting only of Florence Nightingale.

The lady probationers were to be selected by Mrs Wardroper. They were to be between 25 and 35, and had to present a character reference from their family doctor. Abandoned wives who had turned to nursing were not considered. The training of probationers was to last one year and to be completed within that year. Each successful candidate was to receive a certificate. The probationers were paid from the fund, which also supplied them with lodging, tea and sugar, washing and their outer uniform. It was brown, with a white apron and cap. Lady probationers paid up to £52 for the privilege of working a 60-hour week, and ordinary probationers were paid a salary of £8–£20 a year. Mrs Wardroper reported that the 15 probationers were given '1 Alpaca dress and mantle, 2 print ditto, 3 aprons, 3 collars, 3 caps, 1 bonnet, 1 pair galoshes.' Florence Nightingale decreed what was not worn: 'No crinolines, polonaises, hair-pads are to be worn on duty in the hospital.' (A polonaise was a dress consisting of a bodice with a skirt open from the waist downwards.) Each nurse was to have her own sleeping cubicle, and they were not to do any rough domestic work.

The lady-pupils, who paid for their training, became Florence Nightingale's disciples in the nursing reform movement, and as each trained nurse trained others the ripples from the great movement began to spread. Florence Nightingale kept a vigilant eye on the probationers and followed the career of each sister. Finally, her training school 'acted as a clearing house for nursing appointments throughout the country and to many countries overseas'.

She was very positive about the role her sisters and matrons were to play in the world of nursing. In 1867 she wrote to Mary Jones:

> 'The whole reform in nursing both at home and abroad has consisted in this: to take all power over the Nursing out of the hands of the men, and put it into the hands of *one female trained* head and make her responsible for everything (regarding internal management and discipline) being carried out. . . .'

The lady-pupils were segregated from the ordinary probationers and wore special uniforms. At Guy's Hospital these were 'stately black alpaca gowns'. At the Middlesex they 'were arrayed in a dress of violet hue with a small train, three inches in length which swept the floor behind them'.

Within 15 years or so of its foundation the Nightingale school was receiving requests from hospitals all over the world for trained nurses to start new schools. In most cases Florence Nightingale and Mrs Wardroper would select an outstanding sister and send her, with other nurses, to carry out this work. In 1867, for example, a request for nurses came from Australia and, as a result, a Miss Lucy Osburn with five picked nurses was sent out to start a school in the Infirmary in Sydney. By the early 1880s Florence Nightingale was gratified to find that the majority of important hospitals in the British Isles, Canada, the United States, Germany and Sweden were staffed by nurses trained at her school.

Concurrently with the Nightingale Training School, its indefatigable progenitor decided to allocate some of her fund money to the training of midwives. However, owing to a series of unfortunate incidents, of which the main one was an outbreak of puerperal fever, the experiment was not successful and was eventually shelved.

On the other hand, the success of the school encouraged philanthropists, such as William Rathbone, to consult Florence Nightingale as to how best to bring their particular projects to fruition. Rathbone's concerned a system by which the poor could be nursed by trained nurses in their own homes. As Florence had no nurses to spare at the time, she invited Rathbone to set up his own training school for nurses, and this he did, building and equipping a school at the Royal Infirmary, Liverpool.

Workhouse infirmaries

A few years later Rathbone again appealed to Florence Nightingale for help. This time it was to improve the nursing in the workhouse infirmaries, where conditions were so dreadful as to have inspired Charles Dickens to write *Oliver Twist*. Florence Nightingale chose one of her favourite pupils, Agnes Jones, to tackle this task. Miss Jones took with her to the Brownlow Infirmary in May 1865 12 other nurses whose salaries were paid by Rathbone. So successful was this experiment that the principle of using trained nurses in workhouses became the rule in Liverpool, and soon afterwards was taken up in London and other major cities. Sadly, in 1868 Agnes Jones died of typhus contracted during her hospital work, and never saw the results of her labours.

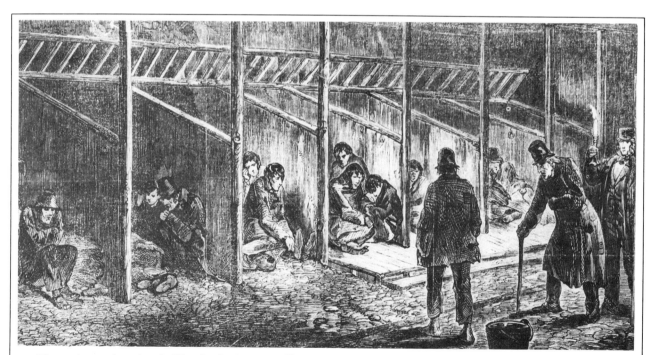

The men's casual ward in the West London Union workhouse c. 1860. Great efforts began to be made about this time to improve conditions in workhouses infirmaries, where there was no proper medical or nursing care.

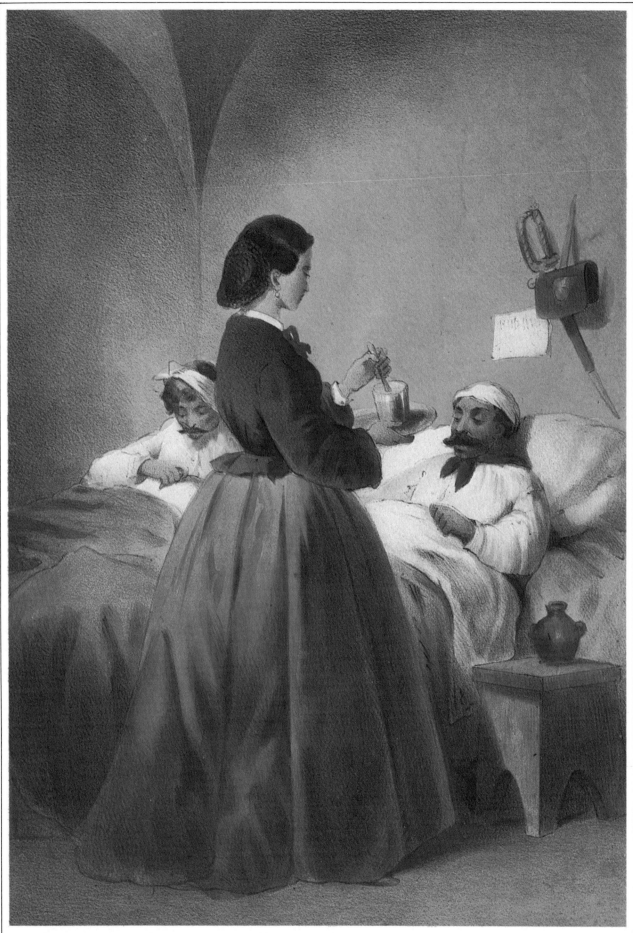

Florence Nightingale administering medicine to soldiers at Scutari Hospital. The reality was much harsher than this somewhat romanticized picture would suggest. Nurses were on their feet for as long as 24 hours at a stretch, dressing wounds, assisting at operations and comforting dying men as best they could.

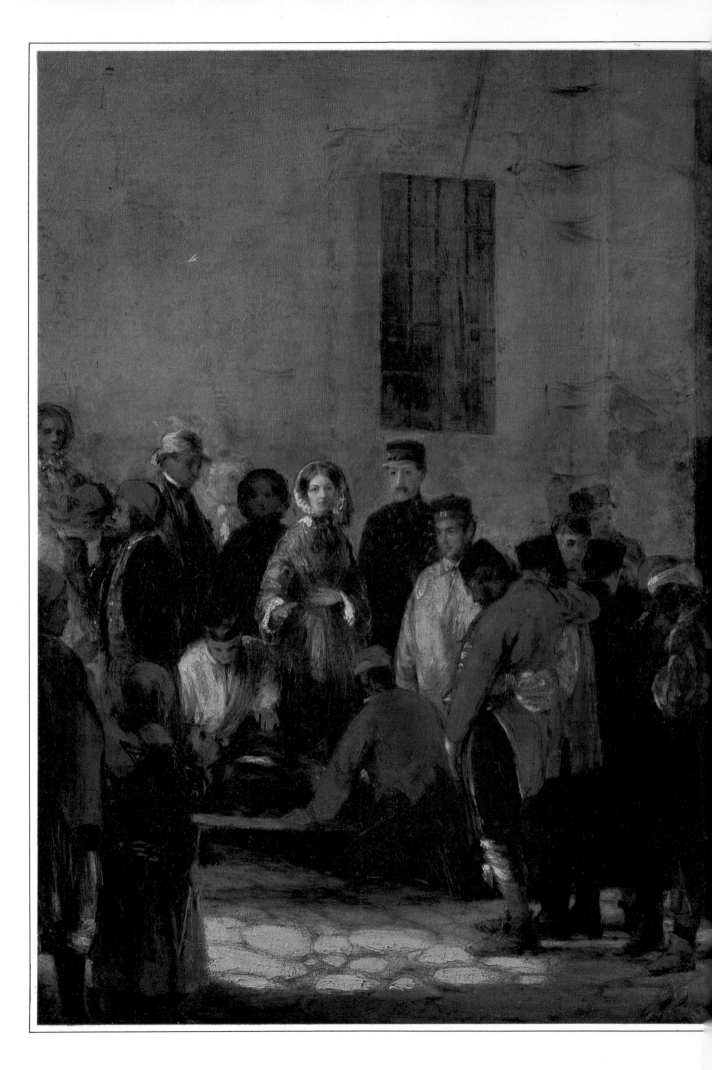

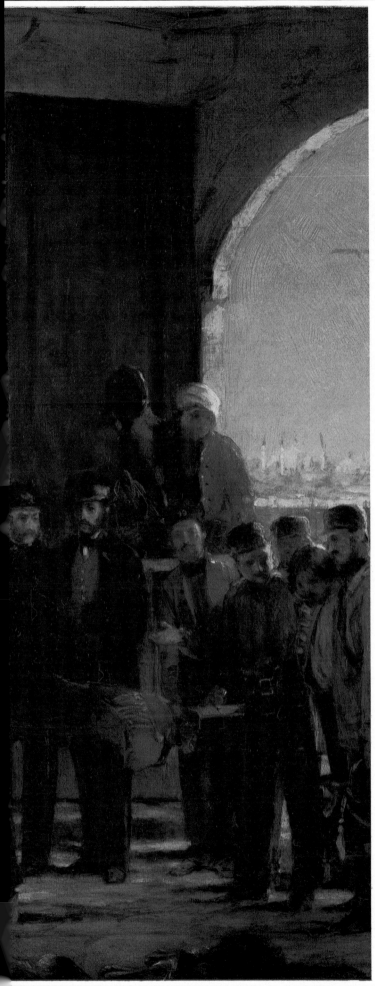

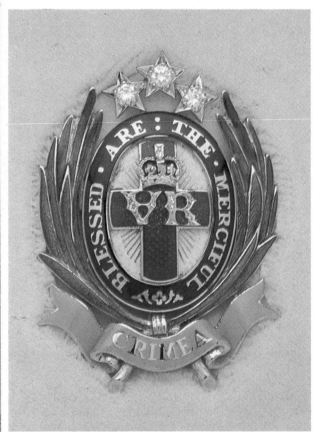

Left *Florence Nightingale at Scutari. Painting by Jerry Barrett, c.1856.*
Above *A replica of the Nightingale Brooch, presented by Queen Victoria to Florence Nightingale in 1856. Throughout her life it remained one of her most cherished possessions.*

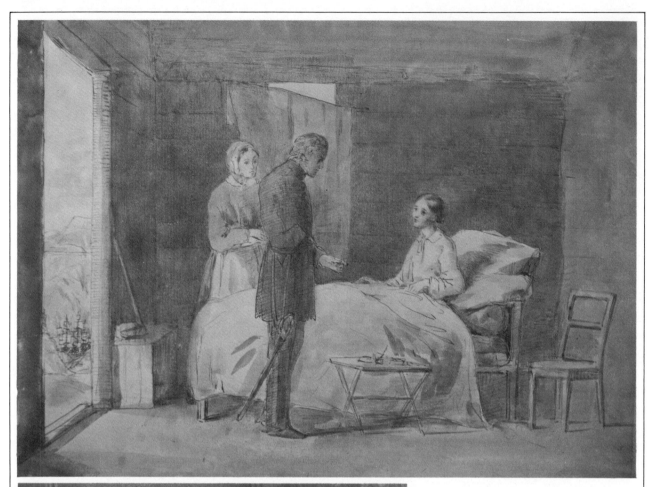

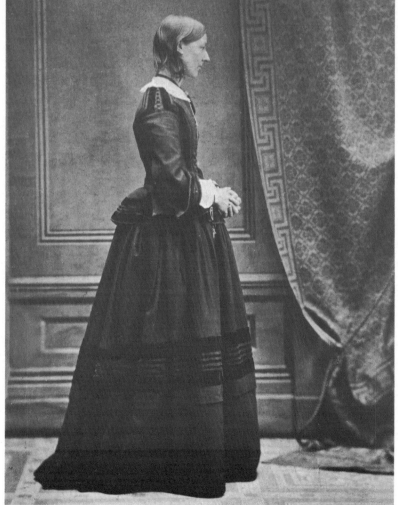

Above *While recovering from a serious illness at Balaclava, in May 1855 Florence Nightingale received a visit from Lord Raglan, the commander-in-chief of the British forces in the Crimea.*
Left *A photograph of Florence Nightingale taken shortly after her return home from the Crimea, exhausted by her Herculean efforts and still physically weak from her recent illness.*

These eventually led to the Metropolitan Poor Law Act which reformed the workhouse infirmaries of London.

Encouraged by Rathbone's interest in district or visiting nursing, Florence Nightingale applied herself to the massive task of founding, in 1875, the Metropolitan and Nursing Association, and chose a Miss F. Lees, one of her best nurses, as its director.

However, much of the credit for the reform of the workhouses and hospitals for the sick and dying must go to Louisa Twining (1820–1911), who dedicated her life to improving conditions in these places. Like Florence Nightingale she came from a wealthy family. Her father was a prosperous London barrister, and her campaign was prompted by a visit she made to an old woman who had been taken to the workhouse in the Strand in London. Louisa Twining was devastated by what she saw there. She noted the insolent porters who restricted visits, the young chronically sick, kept like animals in darkness and filth, and the odious behaviour of the drunken warders and nurses.

Despite great opposition she brought her campaign to the notice of the public, whose conscience was deeply stirred. In 1886 Louise Twining formed an association for trained nurses in workhouses, and later set up a home for epileptic girls which she furnished with her own family furniture. She ran the home herself until well into old age.

Florence Nightingale had given nursing the seal of respectability. Now sweeping reforms and discoveries in medicine were to have far-reaching effects on every aspect of nursing and on midwifery in particular.

Children's hospitals

In 1851, the year of the Great Exhibition, Britain did not possess a single children's hospital. There were already several in Europe, of which France could claim the oldest. L'Hôpital des Enfants Malades, in the Rue de Sèvre, Paris, first opened its doors in 1676 as a foundling hospital and was turned into a hospital for sick children during the Revolution.

In Britain the feverish atmosphere of industrial expansion and the pursuit of wealth had led to the neglect of the needs of sick children. Children were important in so far as they could help the family budget in the fields, in the factories and in the coal mines.

Lord Ashley (later Lord Shaftesbury) was one of the most tireless champions of reforms intended to make the lives of children, both sick and well, easier. He laboured ceaselessly in Parliament for practical legislative action, his efforts leading finally in 1840 to the appointment of the Children's Employment Commission. The Commission's first report, which concerned juvenile labour in coal mines, contained some terrifying facts, including children of seven or eight years working 16 hours a day below ground. The Commission's findings, together with the writings of Dickens,

Kingsley, Carlyle and Disraeli, all urging reform, stirred the public conscience and in 1844 the new Factory Bill became law. It limited the hours of work for children under 14 to six and a half hours a day.

At this time, however, there were no facilities for treating children as in-patients in hospitals. Of the 50,000 deaths occurring annually in London, 21,000 were of children under ten. A number of children were treated at the Royal Universal Dispensary in the Waterloo Road by a Dr Charles West. His main interest was combating disease in children, and a book he wrote on this subject was translated into most known languages. His greatest ambition was to found a hospital which would admit only children. Not everyone thought, as he did, that a hospital was the best place for a very sick child. The widely held belief was that children should be cared for at home by their mothers, since hospitals were hotbeds of infection. In any case hospitals in London did not readily admit sick children. The London Hospital refused 'all children under seven except such as required amputation or cutting for the stone'. At one time Guy's Hospital had had 15 cribs for children located in a wooden building over some stables. In 1850 these were pulled down and not replaced.

Dr West, together with a number of friends, determined to interest the general public in a children's hospital, and such was the enthusiasm for this project that towards the end of the year the Provisional Committee, formed in 1850, was looking around for suitable premises. Long before, Dr West, on one of his strolls through London, had come across what he felt was the 'dream' house for his hospital, in Great Ormond Street, and, finally, through a succession of happy coincidences, on 29 April 1851, a lease for No 49 Great Ormond Street was signed. West's dream became reality and the London Hospital for Sick Children came into being.

The public, and in particular men like Charles Dickens and Lord Shaftesbury, were enthusiastic about the new hospital, whose functions included providing for the reception, maintenance and medical treatment of the children of the poor during sickness and furnishing their mothers with advice. The hospital also aimed to promote the advancement of medical science generally with reference to the diseases of children and, in particular, to provide for the more efficient instruction of students in this department of medical knowledge. In addition it proposed to disseminate among all classes of the community, but chiefly among the poor, a better acquaintance with the management of infants and children during illness by serving as a 'school for the education and training of women in the special duties of children's nursing'.

Great Ormond Street is often known as the mother of children's hospitals, for its example was followed elsewhere, and children's hospitals were started in Norwich, Edinburgh, Glasgow, Manchester, Liverpool, Birmingham, Gloucester and Brighton.

In 1887, in celebration of Queen Victoria's Jubilee, the children of the Empire contributed a large sum which helped

towards the erection of the South Wing facing Great
Ormond Street. The new block was opened by the Prince
and Princess of Wales on 4 June 1893. Further developments
took place when other buildings were incorporated into the
hospital. From time to time through the years additions and
structural alterations were made to keep pace with the
request for more beds and more facilities, and today the
Great Ormond Street Hospital for Sick Children is one of
the most famous children's hospitals in the world.

The advance of medicine

'The nineteenth century was a period of scientific discovery
in medicine which, liberated from Galenic dogmatism,
finally recognized the fundamental truth that anatomical,
physiological and pathological knowledge constituted the
basis of all medical studies and were the basis on which the
whole structure of modern medicine was to be erected.'
(From *History of Medicine* by Arturo Castiglioni, 1941.)

In the early part of the century progress was influenced by
a number of intellectual, political and social currents
prevalent at this time. Public health, for long ignored by
politicians and the medical profession, became a subject of
great importance as urban centres developed and their
inhabitants insisted on better sanitary conditions.

The greatest advances were made in France by such giants
of modern medicine as Pierre Louis, the founder of medical
statistics, René Laennec, the inventor of the stethoscope
and elucidator of thoracic disease, Jean Nicholas Corvisart,
the great expert on diseases of the heart, Philippe Pinel, the
reformer of the asylum, Marie François Bichat, the father
of modern histology, and Pierre Bretonneau, the
epidemiologist.

They were followed by the Austrians who belonged to the
famous Vienna School, including Skoda, the great clinical
expert, Rokitansky, one of the founders of modern pathological anatomy, Hebra, the founder of scientific
dermatology, and Semmelweiss, who introduced antiseptic
methods into midwifery.

In England important clinical and surgical advances were
made by men who, following in the footsteps of the great
John Hunter, made medical history in surgery, anatomy and
physiology. Probably medicine's greatest revolution came
about with the introduction of anaesthesia in the United
States by William Morton, which was later popularized in
Britain in obstetric practice by James Simpson.

Modern medicine and nursing also owe a vast debt to two
men, neither of whom had a medical degree. One was
Charles Darwin who, by placing the doctrine of evolution on
an observational basis, gave a new stimulus and meaning to
all biological research. The other was Louis Pasteur (and
after him Koch and Lister) who by his demonstration of the
germinal origin of pathological processes classified a great
number of previously inexplicable phenomena.

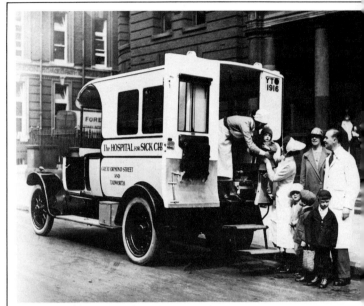

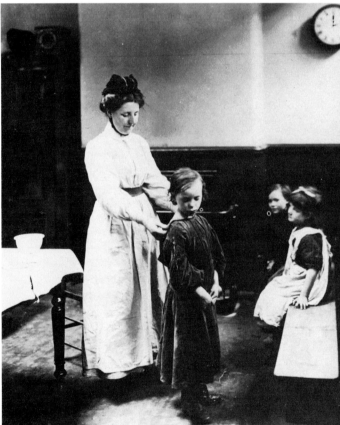

Top *An ambulance standing outside the Hospital for Sick
Children, Great Ormond Street, London, in the late 1920s.*
Above *Medical attention for the young. Children being
examined for lice by a health visitor at a cleansing station in
the early twentieth century.*
Opposite, above *Mark Ward, St Bartholomew's Hospital,
London, in the early twentieth century, with nurses and male
patients both young and old.*
Opposite, below *A scene in a ward in the East London
Hospital for Children in 1878.*

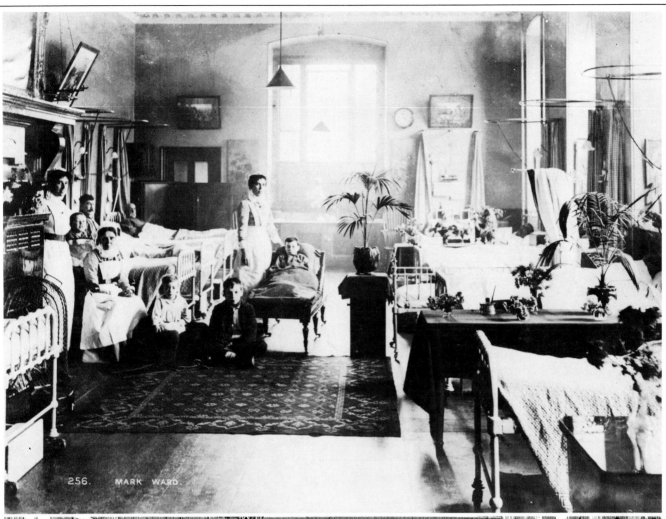

256. MARK WARD.

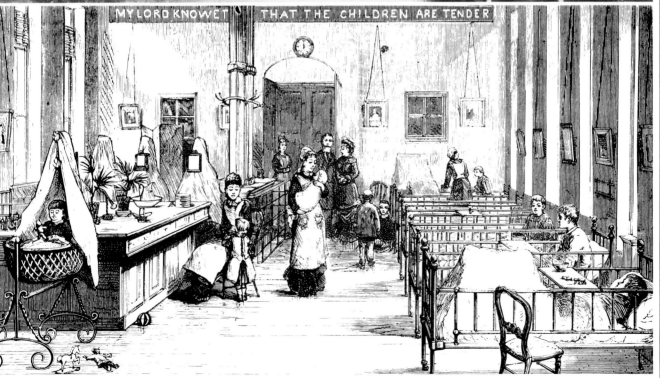

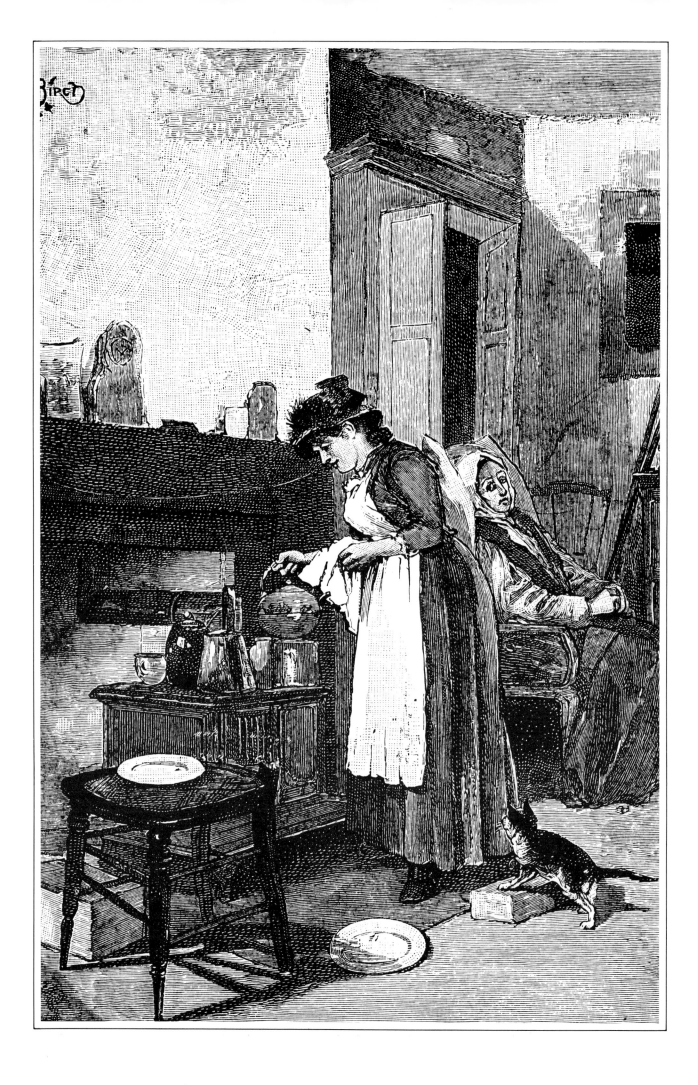

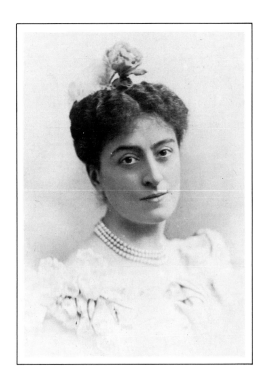

The struggle for registration

Ethel Gordon Manson

In 1881 a young woman of 24, whose influence on the future development of nursing was to be far-reaching, became matron of St Bartholomew's Hospital. Ethel Gordon Manson, one of the new breed of 'lady nurses' was intelligent, spirited and well-educated, and came from a wealthy background. She was also, like Florence Nightingale, a reformer with a great sense of her own importance. She headed a generation of lady nurses who, like herself, felt it was vital to establish some form of distinction between trained and untrained nurses. What they wanted was a state register of nurses which would effectively separate the sheep from the goats.

Ethel Gordon Manson and her friends were substantially correct in feeling that urgent reforms in the system of nursing were needed. They were also aware that the standards in the training schools varied widely. London hospitals had higher standards than those of the less well endowed regional hospitals, which, being unable to provide more rigorous courses of training, used cheap labour in the form of probationers.

Top *Ethel Gordon Manson, later Mrs Ethel Bedford Fenwick, who devoted much of her life to the struggle to secure state registration for nurses. She was also a noted suffragette.*
Opposite *A nurse visiting a sick woman in a tenement house. District nursing began in Liverpool in the early 1860s under the auspices of William Rathbone, a wealthy philanthropist. Illustration from* Century Magazine, *1882.*

A state register, said Ethel Gordon Manson, would do as much to protect the interests of patients as those of the nurses themselves. This was an interesting, even revolutionary, concept. Until the advent of Florence Nightingale the views and physical comfort of the patient had not been rated particularly highly by either the medical faculty or the nurses, since the *health* of the invalid, not his welfare or creature comforts, had always been their prime concern.

The principal aim of registration was to guarantee that no nurse considered unfit could register or, in the event of her having registered and been found wanting, that her name could be instantly removed. The only stumbling block was the definition of a 'qualified' nurse. It was felt that training alone was not a sufficient test, for many hospitals issued certificates, even though the quality of their training was debatable. It was thought that the best solution to this particular problem was to set up a central body which would be empowered to make the all-important decision. Furthermore, there should be a national examination to ascertain whether each individual trainee had obtained sufficient benefit from her course, only those who had passed this examination qualifying for admission to the register.

Florence Nightingale was horrified at the idea of registration. So far as she was concerned nursing was and always would be an art and a vocation. 'Nursing is an art,' she wrote, 'and if it is to be made an art, requires as exclusive a devotion, as hard a preparation, as any painter's or sculptor's work; for what is the having to do with dead canvas or cold marble compared with having to do with the living body – the temple of God's spirit. It is one of the Arts; I had almost said, the finest of the Fine Arts.'

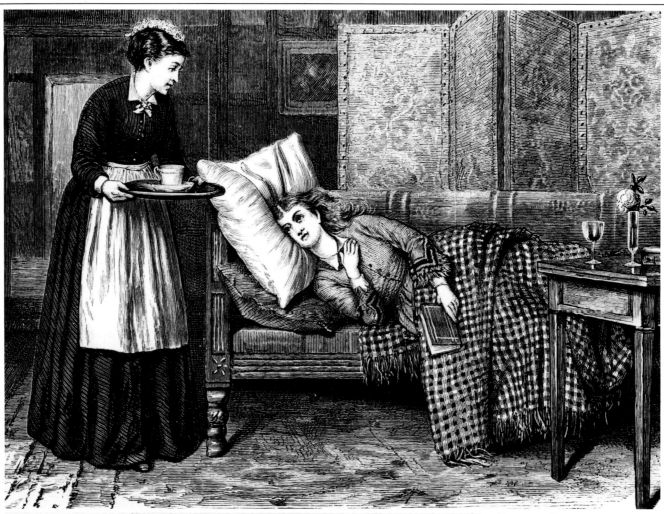

Letter from Miss FLORENCE NIGHTINGALE.

Dec 16/96

10, SOUTH STREET,
PARK LANE, W.

Dear Duke of Westminster
   Good speed to your noble effort in favour of 'District Nurses' for town "& country"; and in Commemoration of our Queen who cares for all.
   We look upon the District Nurse, if she is what she should be, & if we give her the training she should have, as the Great civilizer of the poor: training as well as nursing them out of ill health into good health (Health Missioners), out of drink into self control, but all without preaching, without patronizing — as friends in Sympathy.
   But let them hold the Standard high as Nurses
   Pray be sure, I will try to help all I can, tho' that be small, here I will with your leave let you know.
   Pray believe me your Grace's faithful Servant
   Florence Nightingale

Opposite, above *A visiting nurse wearing a 'fever-proof' costume. Despite the advances in medicine in the nineteenth century the risk of infection from a number of contagious diseases remained considerable.*
Opposite, below *District nurses in uniform. The concept of nursing people in their own homes was to prove remarkably successful. Illustration from Girls' Own Paper, 1877.*
Above *'The Invalid'. In the nineteenth century many of the simpler nursing duties could be carried out by domestic servants.*
Left *A letter to the Duke of Westminster from Florence Nightingale on the subject of district nursing.*

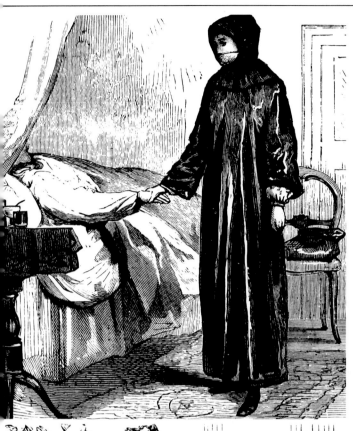

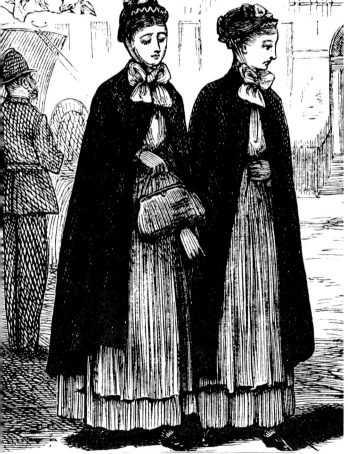

Florence Nightingale had not changed her views about country girls making the best nurses, but this belief was not endorsed by Ethel Gordon Manson and her friends. They saw training as a period of initiation, a kind of 'ordeal by fire' to test the physical, moral, spiritual and intellectual powers of the trainee. They believed that the best nursing material would have to be selected from young women from the middle class, and that the choice of these nurses would rest equally on their educational background and financial independence.

Unmoved by Florence Nightingale's reactions to the idea of registration, Ethel Gordon Manson stuck to her guns and pressed on with her campaign. By now the young matron had married a wealthy doctor and, as Mrs Bedford Fenwick, gave up nursing and concentrated on founding a salon which would further the cause of registration, as well as helping along the crusade of her close friend, the suffragette Emmeline Pankhurst.

In fact, the motivations of Mrs Bedford Fenwick and her allies were not entirely altruistic. They were, for the most part, ardent feminists and, in seeking to enhance their own status, they were also hoping to strike a blow for women's rights. 'The nurse question is the woman question,' said Mrs Bedford Fenwick, who also felt that it was important to work on terms of equality with the medical profession and acquire a stronger voice in hospital administration and management.

Florence Nightingale continued to oppose all her reforms. Registration, she said, would involve examinations for nurses. Although these might show them to have a retentive mind for book learning, in her view no examination could possibly produce the kind of nurse for whom she had laid down training and who could be the only kind of nurse to meet with her approval.

The battle continued to rage. Although Florence Nightingale led a retired and cloistered life, she was in constant touch with people in high places and very soon and very forcefully communicated to them her views on registration. They, in their turn, made their disapproval known. Sydney Holland, like Florence Nightingale, a governor of the London Hospital, was loud in his condemnation of Mrs Bedford Fenwick's reforms:

> 'We want to stop nurses thinking themselves anything more than they are, namely the faithful carriers out of the doctor's orders. The other side are always talking about nursing being a profession, and 'graduates' in nursing just as they do in America.' (*Select Committee on Registration 1905*, p. 37)

Miss Hughes, the superintendent of a nursing association, was vociferous in her support of Florence Nightingale's views on what made a good nurse:

> I know that some of the most successful medical nurses are those who had been upper servants, that they fitted into households, caused less jar and

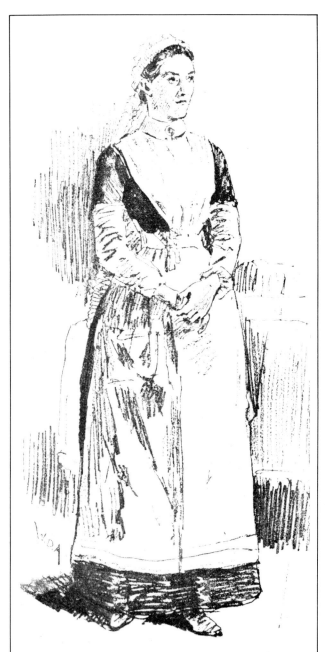

A nursing sister in 1888. By the latter part of the nineteenth century nursing was well established as a respectable profession.

friction than many of those who considered themselves superior in station, who could not adapt themselves so well.' (*Select Committee on Registration 1905*, p. 84.)

The Royal British Nurses' Association

Despite tremendous opposition from many quarters Mrs Bedford Fenwick and her supporters continued their struggle, and finally the British Nurses' Association came into being in 1887 with Mrs Bedford Fenwick as permanent president, and the other nurse-founders as permanent vice-presidents. The British Nurses' Association (from 1901 the Royal British Nurses' Association) was declared 'a union of nurses for professional objects', containing, according to the president and her friends, 'the elite of the profession'.

It soon became clear that the newly formed association had considerable influence and formed a powerful pressure group in favour of state registration. While waiting for official sanction, it opened its own register, to which were admitted up to 1 Jan. 1889, those nurses who produced 'satisfactory evidence of professional attainments and personal character and of having been engaged three years in nursing'.

In 1893 Mrs Bedford Fenwick bought the *Nursing Record*, renamed the *British Journal of Nursing*. For over 50 years this forceful and determined woman was to be the editor of her magazine, which she and her supporters used as their mouthpiece. Also, much to the aggravation of Florence Nightingale's followers, the president of the RBNA managed to persuade Queen Victoria's daughter, Princess Christian, to be their patron.

Quietly Florence Nightingale frustrated the move by the RBNA to get registration through by means of an Act of Parliament. The alternative was to apply for a Royal Charter, by which it would be entitled to register nurses. This application led to an enquiry held by the Privy Council in 1893, and a Charter was granted. However, the power asked for included the word 'register'. In the power granted the word 'list' had been substituted for 'register', thus entirely evading the point at issue. Exactly as Florence Nightingale had wished, the RBNA's list had no control over the training schools and very few nurses were interested in putting their names on it.

Although popular among her friends and admirers, Mrs Bedford Fenwick was both aggressive and self-opinionated. The result was that she made so many enemies that in 1894 she had the humiliation of being voted off the council of the RBNA which had been her brain-child. Her husband, who had been treasurer, immediately resigned and, to add to her mortification, registration was dropped by the RBNA.

Nevertheless, Mrs Bedford Fenwick was still to achieve some impressive results which ensured her an honoured place in the history of nursing. In 1893 she went to the United States to attend the Chicago World Fair, at which there was a British Nurses' Stand organized by her. At the fair she met the superintendents of a large number of American nurse-training schools, most of which were modelled on either Nightingale or Kaiserswerth principles.

The American women were much taken with Mrs Bedford Fenwick's personality and ideas and, as a result of their meeting with her, formed their own Society of Superintendents of Training Schools. She also met the then president of the International Council of Women, and was inspired to form in 1900 the International Council of Nurses on the same lines. She had already formed the Matrons' Council of Great Britain and Ireland, and in 1904 created the National Council of Nurses to represent British nurses on the International Council.

Her new campaign had been strengthened in 1902 by the passing of the Midwives Act, the final result of bills presented to Parliament since 1878. After this Act became law no woman could attend women in childbirth otherwise than under the direction of a qualified practitioner, unless she was certified under the Act. Certification and registration were to be the responsibility of a Central Midwives Board, consisting of five doctors, and five other persons, one to be appointed by the RBNA. Qualification was one year in bona-fide practice and a certificate of good character. This had been backed by both the General Medical Council and the Royal College of Physicians, who were divided on the subject of registration of nurses as distinct from midwives.

Finally, however, in 1905 a Select Committee was appointed to report on the matter of registration, and found in its favour:

'It is desirable that a Register of Nurses should be kept by a Central Body organized by the State, and that while it is not desirable to prohibit unregistered persons for nursing for gain, no person should be entitled to assume the title "Registered Nurse", whose name is *not* upon the Register.'

The central body was to approve training schools and to admit to the Register those who had appropriate training, were equipped with the requisite knowledge and experience, and were of good character.

As soon as the Select Committee had reported in favour of registration, the nursing organizations made a vociferous call for prompt action, and every year, from 1904 to 1914, a registration bill was presented to Parliament. Mrs Bedford Fenwick haunted the lobby of the House of Commons, 'instructing, persuading, pleading', but to no avail. The dispute dragged on into the early years of the twentieth century without a solution.

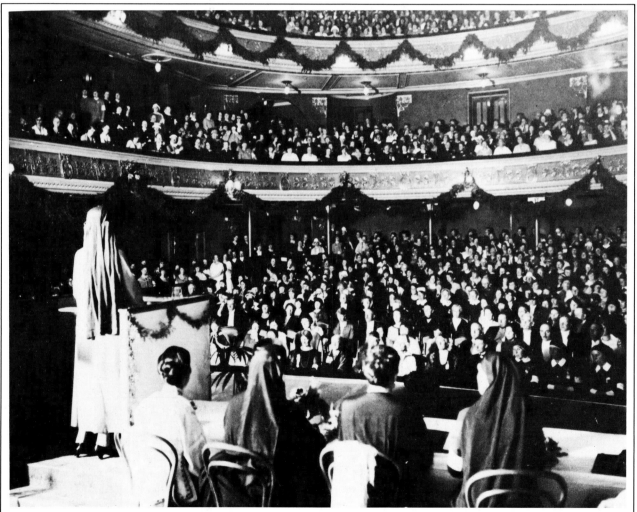

A meeting of the International Council of Nurses in Helsinki in 1925. The council had been established in London in 1899, holding its first congress at Buffalo, New York, in 1901.

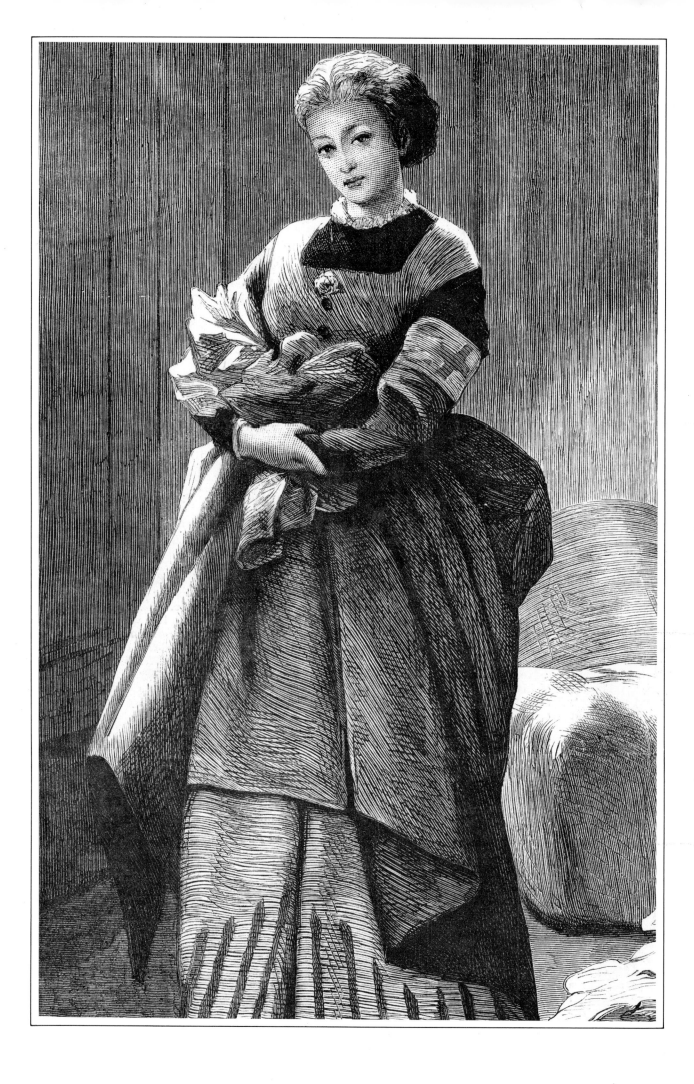

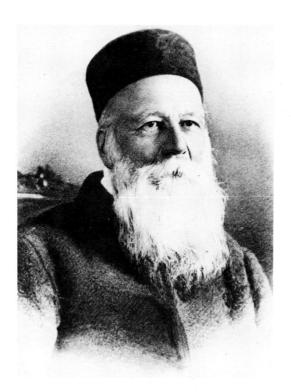

Red Cross, army, navy and air force nursing

The origins of the Red Cross

In April 1859 Austria declared war against France and Italy. The ensuing campaign was short and violent, and was to have far-reaching future consequences for fighting men everywhere. It was the bloody aftermath of the Battle of Solferino, fought on 24 June 1859, that was to make a young Swiss industrialist, Jean Henri Dunant, world famous.

Dunant, the son of a wealthy Swiss merchant, was a sensitive, idealistic young man, much addicted to good works. But on the day of the battle his only thought was to secure the patronage of the Emperor Napoleon III in a land development venture in Algeria in which he was interested. Having sought for months in vain to get an interview with the emperor, Dunant decided that the war in Italy might provide an opportunity, since Napoleon III was known to be constantly with his troops.

Dunant was something of an exquisite and, wearing a

Top *Jean Henri Dunant, the Swiss philanthropist and founder of the Red Cross. Dunant's book,* A Memory of Solferino, *published in 1862, made a great impact and the first voluntary relief services were set up in the following year.*
Opposite *A Red Cross nurse in 1870. After the establishment of the International Red Cross in 1864, national societies were formed in a number of European countries.*

stylish white tropical suit, he left Geneva and made for the Apennine village of Pontremoli. Here he found an influential friend who gave him a letter of recommendation to the French general, MacMahon, adding: 'If you want to see a first-class battle you should cross the Apennines at once.'

Dunant's destination was Napoleon's headquarters at Castiglione, which he reached on the morning of the 24th. He was almost immediately engulfed by a torrent of wounded who lay about in the burning sun without water or care of any kind. Dunant was appalled, and immediately set about organizing help.

He set up his first-aid station in the Church of San Maggiore, where '500 men, Frenchmen, Arabs, Germans, their faces black with flies lay together.' Four Austrian doctors, a German physician and two Italian students did their utmost to help the injured and the dying. Dunant, in his crisp white suit, was indefatigable. He had implored the help of the women of the town, who willingly brought water for the men and helped to wash their wounds. Then he rounded up a number of tourists – English, French and Italians – to dress wounds, carry messages and write letters for the dying.

Dunant's mission of mercy went on for weeks and, when he finally returned home to Geneva, he was haunted by the sufferings of the men he had tried to help. His nerves were shattered, and he became restless and irritable. He knew he had to let the world know what he had seen and experienced on the battlefield. Finally he sat down at his desk . . . 'In writing *A Memory of Solferino*,' he said, 'I was, as it were, lifted out of myself, compelled by some higher power, and inspired by the breath of God.'

Dunant's book was published in the autumn of 1862. Copies were sent to reigning monarchs, princes, and ministers of war and foreign affairs. It caused a sensation, and Dunant received letters of encouragement from such people as Victor Hugo, Charles Dickens and Ernest Renan. He had, he was told, written a book that would stir consciences and bring about much needed help to war victims. However, Florence Nightingale, one of Dunant's heroines, was as unmoved by his book as were the French military authorities, who condemned it as being a thoroughly exaggerated work of fantasy.

Although *A Memory of Solferino* had made a tremendous impact, its message might soon have been forgotten, had it not been for the drive and persistence of Gustave Moynier, one of Geneva's leading lawyers. He was so impressed by Dunant's book that he suggested that the subject of aid for wounded soldiers should be discussed at a meeting of the Genevese Society for Public Welfare, of which he was chairman. This historic meeting took place on 9 Feb. 1863. On the agenda appeared an item: 'Proposal (as set out in *A Memory of Solferino*) to form during a time of peace and tranquillity, relief societies whose aim should be to help the wounded in time of war by means of volunteers, zealous, devoted and well-qualified for such a work.' Thus was the stage set for the founding of the International Red Cross.

At a conference on 8 Aug. 1864, attended by representatives from 26 countries, the Geneva Convention was accepted. It laid down certain principles to be observed in war: the wounded were to be respected; military hospitals were to be neutral; and medical personnel were to be protected. The symbol of the Red Cross, an inversion of the Swiss flag, was adopted. The provisions of the Convention were later extended to the crews of ships at sea.

The British Red Cross Society was founded in 1870 to tend the sick and wounded in war and alleviate distress in peace. The Society is autonomous and independent, but adheres to the rules of the International Red Cross. In peacetime it carries on first aid, auxiliary nursing, and other welfare activities. In war it supplements the medical services of the Crown, and provides amenities which fall outside the scope of official provisions.

In 1888 the Royal Red Cross was founded by Queen Victoria, the award being given in two classes. Those in the first class were known as members and those in the second as associates. The award was restricted to women in the nursing service, or to women who had displayed outstanding qualities in the care of the sick and the wounded of the fighting services. The Royal Red Cross was awarded at once to two Crimean nurses, Florence Nightingale and Sister Mary Aloysius.

The American Red Cross came into being in 1881 mainly through the efforts of Clara Barton (1821–1912), its first

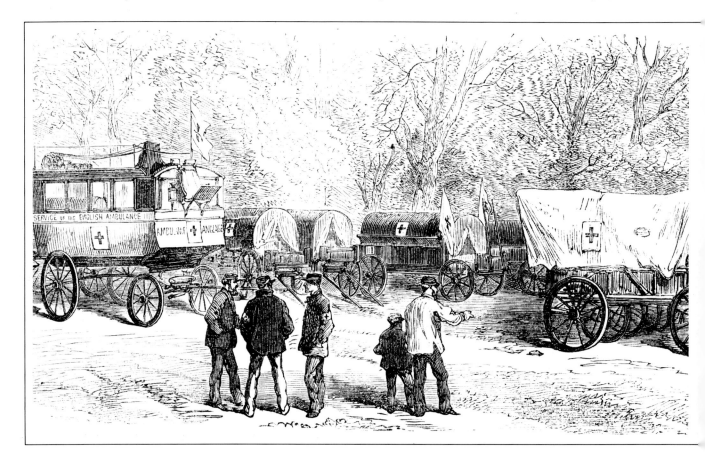

president. Known as 'The angel of the battlefield', Clara Barton virtually acted as unpaid quartermaster to the wounded of the American Civil War. An almost exact contemporary of Florence Nightingale, she resembled her not only in her work in time of war, but in her refusal to allow poor health to prevent her carrying on with her duties until she was well into her eighties. In 1882 the United States became a member of the International Red Cross, and soon after instituted the Red Cross Nursing Service, which is the reserve of the Army and Navy Nurse Corps.

Early in the Civil War, Dorothea Dix, who had been engaged upon important work to improve conditions in prisons, poorhouses and mental hospitals, was appointed Superintendent of Female Nurses for the Army. At that time ward masters and orderlies helped with the nursing in hospitals, while the women nurses dressed wounds, gave medicine, and attended to diets. The value of trained nurses was proved by the Spanish-American War (1898–9), when about 1500 trained nurses gave valuable help.

The St John Ambulance Association

The St John Ambulance Association was founded in 1877 to provide first-aid training and to supply ambulance material. Its teaching was intended to reach all parts of the community, and within six months of its establishment there were 12 registered association centres, through which over 1000 people had received instruction in first aid. As early as 1903 proposals were made for the formation of a junior organization and eventually the Cadet branch was established in 1922 to provide teaching in first aid and nursing and involvement in community services and adventure training.

Army nursing

In every country with a Red Cross organization there is during war some connection between this organization and the official military nursing service, where such exists, although the rules governing this connection vary from country to country. Few countries have military nurses, employing only nurses attached to military hospitals. Few of these nurses are actually trained in military hospitals. A number of countries call for help from the Red Cross nursing personnel for military duties only in war, and have regular permanent services for female nurses for the armed forces. These nurses must all be state-registered before they begin their government work and also have to undergo a special examination or a period of probation. Military nurses wear military uniform when on duty, and in nearly all countries have relative rank or official status. Canada was the first country to give rank to its military nurses. In July 1904, when the Canadian Army Medical Corps was reorganized, arrangements were made for 25 nursing sisters with the rank and allowances of lieutenants.

After the Crimean War, in Britain a few women nurses were appointed to military hospitals, but most of the nursing was carried out by the men of the Army Hospital Corps, which had just been created. A proposal to increase the number of women nurses employed in military hospitals came before the Financial Secretary to the War Office in Benjamin Disraeli's government in 1877. The scheme had been initiated in 1861 at the Royal Herbert Hospital, Woolwich. This was an important innovation, achieved only after long and earnest pleading by Florence Nightingale, in the face of determined official scepticism and opposition. The Financial Secretary heartily endorsed the plan for increasing the numbers of women nurses, and the first superintendent was one of Florence Nightingale's nurses from the Crimea. The experiment was so successful that it was extended to the Royal Victoria Hospital, Netley, where the nursing was taken over by a Mrs Jane Deeble and six ward sisters from St Thomas' Hospital.

In 1880 the British Red Cross Society decided to use part of the interest accruing from its invested capital to initiate some kind of peacetime work. Women nurses from the Royal Victoria Hospital had given valuable service in South Africa during the Zulu War, and the Society asked the War Office for permission to train a small number of women nurses who would be available for service in any future emergency. A

The Franco-German war of 1870–1 provided the newly formed British Red Cross with an opportunity to prove its usefulness, and surgeons and nurses tended the wounded on both sides. **Left** *An English Red Cross volunteer who served in Saarbrucken.* **Far left** *An English ambulance train encamped near Paris. Illustrated London News, 1870/1.*

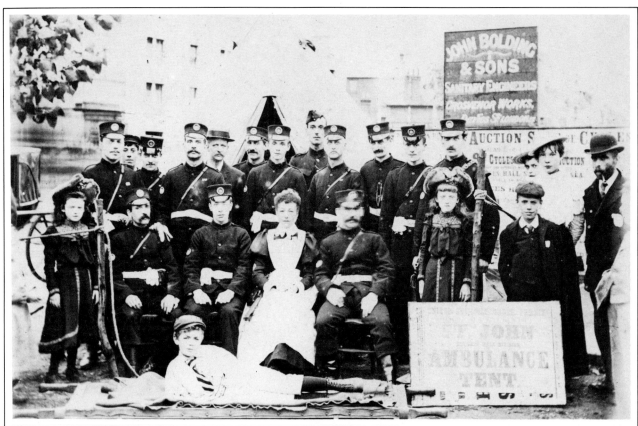

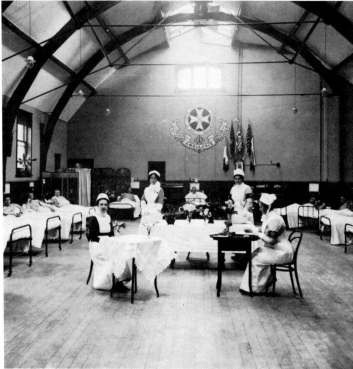

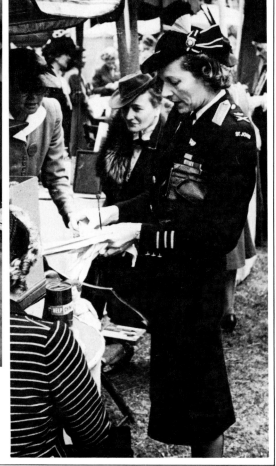

Top *Members of the St John Ambulance Association at the turn of the century.*
Above *A VAD hospital in Rochdale, Lancashire, during the First World War.*
Right *Lady Mountbatten, always a tireless worker on behalf of the Red Cross and the St John Ambulance Brigade.*

favourable reply was received and in May 1881 eight young women reported for duty at Netley. In this way the Society played its part in establishing the principle that women nurses should form part of the staff of service hospitals at home and overseas.

In 1881 an Army Nursing Service was founded, and in 1888 the rule that a staff of sisters was to be appointed to every military hospital of 100 beds and over was extended to the Indian Army. Three years later it was decided that all sisters must receive previous training in a civil hospital since, until that time, the lady superintendent at Netley had trained all the staff.

In 1901 Queen Alexandra, the beautiful, deaf and unpunctual wife of Edward VII, sent for Sydney Holland, the chairman of the London Hospital, to discuss the reorganization of nursing in the army. Nursing had always been one of her greatest interests and she told him that her aim was to see a really efficient service with herself as its head. She invited him to produce a plan for such a service in consultation with the hero of the South African War, Lord Roberts.

Since an Army Nursing Service already existed with the autocratic Princess Christian as its head, after a great many delicate negotiations, Princess Christian, albeit unwillingly, gave way to the queen, whose Imperial Military Nursing Service was established in 1902 under the control of a Nursing Board, with the queen as president. Alexandra was delighted and personally devised the badge to be worn by QAIMNS nurses – a cross borne on the royal arms of Denmark, surmounted by an imperial crown, and the cipher 'A' within the cross.

Serious difficulties arose, however, when the newly formed Territorial Army wished to have its own nursing service and nursing reserve. Since the Territorial Army had come into being through its 'onlie begetter', the Secretary of State for War, Lord Haldane, he wanted his very capable sister, Elizabeth Haldane, to take over the responsibility of establishing a Territorial Army Nursing Reserve. For four years so many obstacles appeared that it was impossible to put her scheme into action. Queen Alexandra refused to allow the formation of a separate and special nursing service for the Territorial Army with an independent president: 'This, I regret to say, I cannot agree to. I am President of all Military, and Naval Hospitals and Nurses, and at my death the whole concern will pass into the hands of my dear daughter-in-law, so as always to be kept together and under one head.'

Finally, however, all the difficulties were smoothed out and Queen Alexandra kept to herself the presidency of both the Nursing Board of the regular army and the Advisory Council of the Territorial Army Nursing Service.

The queen also took a great interest in the Red Cross as the voluntary body concerned with military nursing. Here too she encountered problems. When her husband came to the throne the affairs of the Red Cross were in a state of confusion. The National Aid Society, to which the queen, as Princess of Wales, had allied herself at the time of the

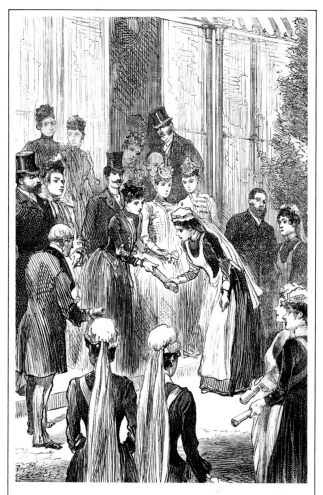

The Princess of Wales (later Queen Alexandra), who always displayed a keen interest in nursing matters, presenting certificates to nurses at Marlborough House, London.
Illustrated London News, 1890.

Sudan campaign, was treated as the British Red Cross by the International Red Cross in Geneva. However, in 1899 a Central British Red Cross Committee had been founded, its object being 'to maintain among voluntary aid societies in time of peace an organization which will render prompt and efficient service in time of war to the sick and wounded, in the manner best suited to supplement the Army Medical Service.'

Thus, relations between this committee and the National Aid Society were more than strained. Eventually it was decided that only intervention at a very high level could break the deadlock between the two Red Cross societies. After consultation with the king and the queen, it was decided that the various bodies concerned with Red Cross work throughout Britain and the British Empire should be amalgamated into one body, to be called the British Red Cross Society, the king to be its patron, and the queen its president. The queen herself in fact presided over the first council meeting, held at Buckingham Palace.

Nursing in the Royal Navy

The Royal Navy has always cared for its sick. The first mention of the obligation to look after sick seamen appears in the Laws of Oleron, sometimes known as the Judgments of Oleron. Dating from around 1194, they were introduced into England by Richard I, and were themselves based on a code of conduct founded by the Republic of Rhodes and adopted by the Romans and other maritime powers of the Mediterranean.

Although many of the laws were harsh, others were more compassionate. One of them required the master of a vessel to put a sick mariner ashore, seek a lodging for him, provide him with a candle of tallow and one of the ship's boys to tend him, or failing that, a hired woman.

In medieval times sick mariners left to fend for themselves ashore were hard pressed to find a bed. The houses of pity, run by monks of various religious orders, usually gave them shelter, but except for the two London hospitals of St Bartholomew's and St Thomas' sick and invalided seamen had no recourse but to find an institution of a religious order.

The increasing use of hospital ships in the seventeenth century marked a greater commitment towards the sick by the naval authorities, who had not always been anxious to foot the hospital bills incurred by their sick mariners. The nurses on board were frequently women, either wives or widows of seamen, but their status was never defined or put on an established basis. When Haslar Hospital, Gosport, and Stonehouse Hospital, Plymouth, opened, women were again used on the wards, coming to the work without any training, since none was available.

Men frequently smuggled females on board ships by the most devious methods and these women were often present during many naval engagements, when they served as nurses to the wounded. Expressions such as 'show a leg' and 'son of a gun' came into use. The former was derived from the custom of allowing women an extra half-hour in their hammocks when the hands were called for morning duties. 'Son of a gun', on the other hand, was the name given to any baby born in a man-of-war. Any woman finding herself in labour was taken below to the main gun deck, where her child was born.

At the outbreak of the Crimean War the Royal Navy despatched to the base hospital at Therapia, Constantinople, a Mrs Eliza Mackenzie with a team of six experienced nursing sisters – the first to be employed by the Royal Navy. The experiment was considered to be a success, and 'full appreciation' was expressed for the work Eliza Mackenzie and for the 'unwearied exertions' of her nurses.

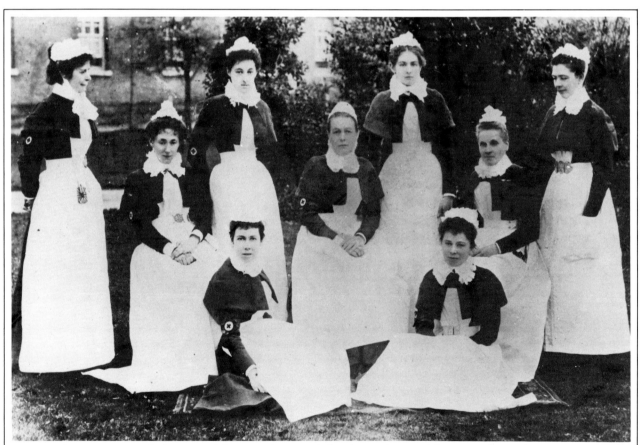

Naval nursing sisters at the beginning of the twentieth century before the introduction of the new uniform and insignia in 1902, when the organization became Queen Alexandra's Royal Naval Nursing Service.

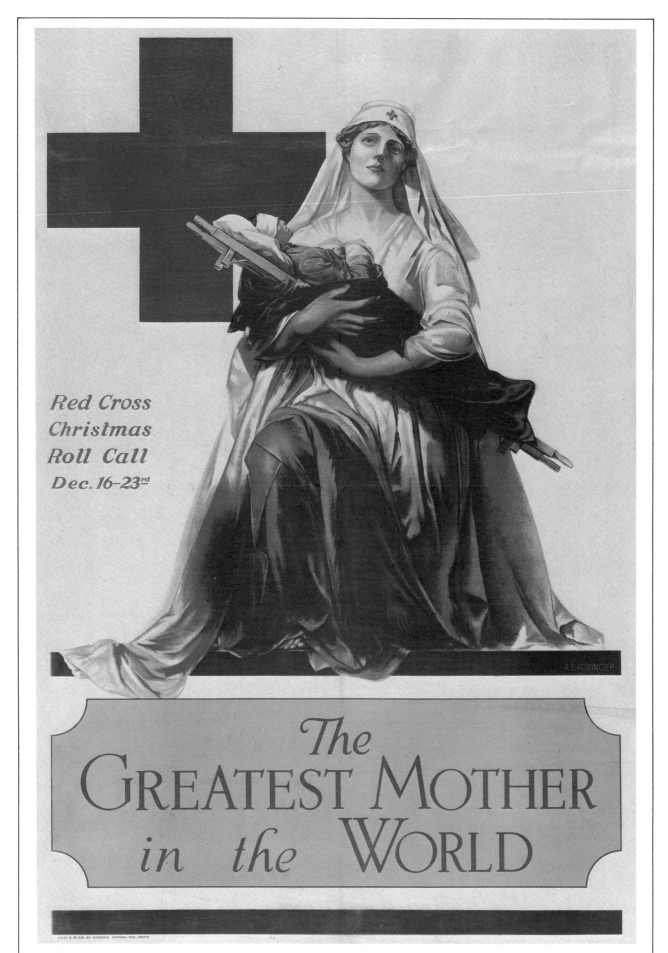

Red Cross
Christmas
Roll Call
Dec. 16-23rd

The
GREATEST MOTHER
in the WORLD

A Red Cross poster from the First World War. In a conflict in which women played an increasingly active role alongside their menfolk, they could still be portrayed as archetypal mother figures, embracing suffering humanity in the form of a wounded soldier.

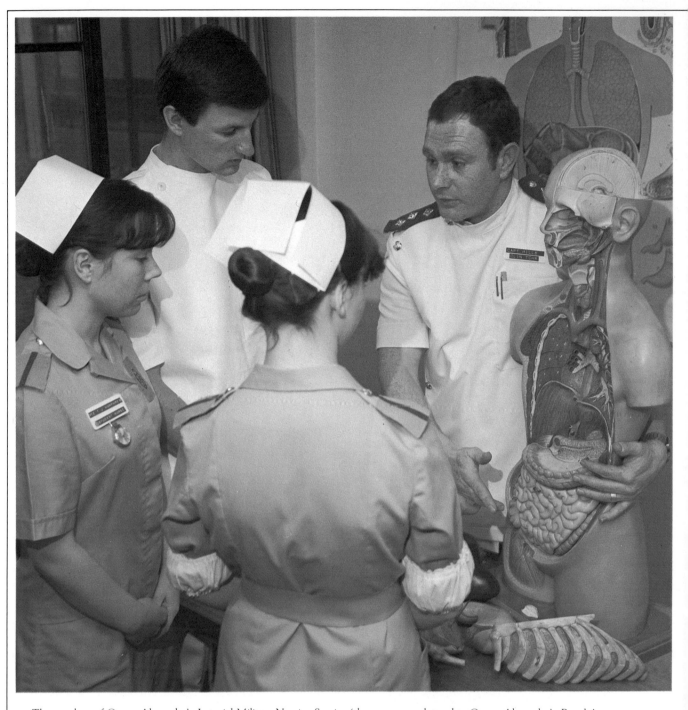

The members of Queen Alexandra's Imperial Military Nursing Service (the name was changed to Queen Alexandra's Royal Army Nursing Corps in 1949) played a distinguished part in both world wars, serving in many parts of the world.
Above *Student nurses undergoing training at the Queen Elizabeth Military Hospital, Woolwich.*
Opposite *A student nurse attending a patient at the Cambridge Military Hospital, Aldershot.*

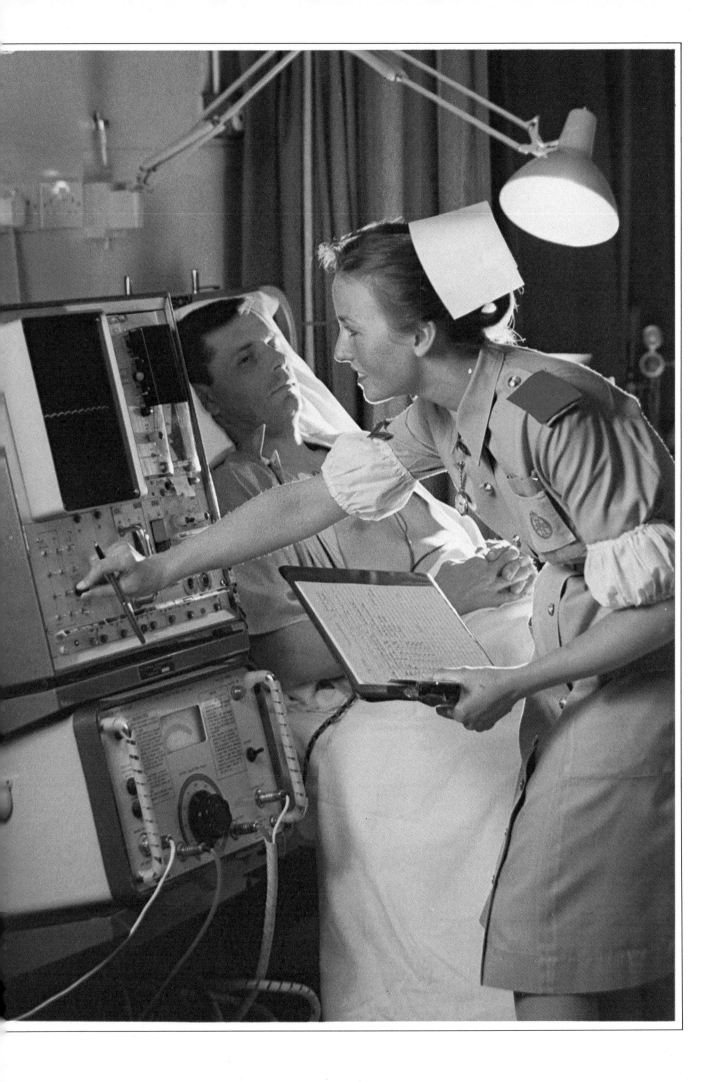

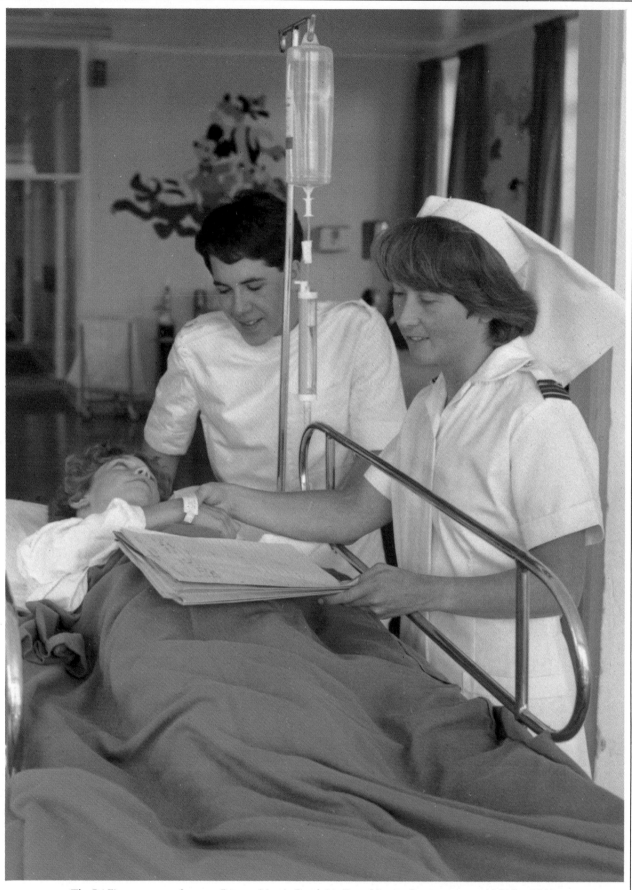

The RAF's own corps of nurses, Princess Mary's Royal Air Force Nursing Service, was established in 1918.
Above *A PMRAFNS nursing officer and a male nurse with a patient. In 1980 the RAF created a unified nursing service, including both male and female nurses.*

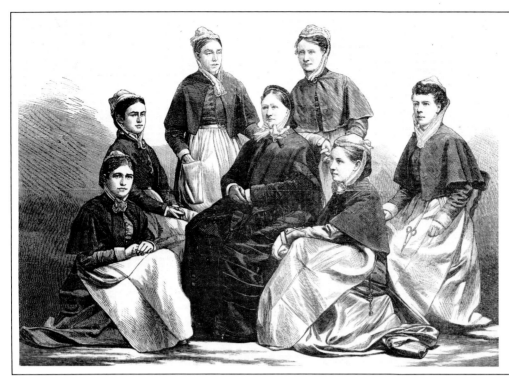

Mrs Jane Deeble, who took charge of nursing at the Royal Victoria Hospital, Netley, and subsequently led a group of nurses to South Africa during the Zulu War of 1879.

The work of Florence Nightingale in the Crimea threw the whole subject of nursing into sharp focus, and a committee was eventually formed to enquire into the organization and training of the sick berth staff of the navy and the nursing staff of the naval hospitals. Known as the Hoskins Committee from the name of its chairman, the committee met in June 1883 and paid visits to all naval and military hospitals. Naval surgeons and sick berth ratings were interviewed and separate opinions were sought from 'thirty experienced naval medical officers', concerning the employment of women in naval hospitals. At the same time the committee sought the advice of Mrs Deeble, superintendent of female staff at the Military Hospital at Netley in Hampshire.

Whether Mrs Deeble influenced the decision of the committee is not known, but the official verdict was favourable, so far as employing women in naval hospitals was concerned. 'We are convinced that a trained female nursing staff is of the highest value to the sick and wounded and there is every reason to believe that nothing but good will result from its introduction.' Thus originated both the idea of trained sick berth ratings and a trained female nursing service.

At the beginning of Oct. 1884 a head sister and six sisters joined Haslar Hospital, while three sisters arrived at Stonehouse. Apart from their general nursing duties, working under the direction of the medical officers the sisters helped in the training of the newly instituted Sick Berth Attendance Branch of the Royal Navy. Reports referred to 'their professional knowledge and skill' and to the fact that their mere presence had a 'humanizing influence' on the patients.

The numbers in the service gradually increased, and in 1900 stood at 29. Sisters were appointed during these years not only to Haslar and Stonehouse but to Melville Hospital, Chatham, the marine infirmaries in Portsmouth and Plymouth, and the Hospital for Lunatics at Yarmouth. They also served in the smaller hospitals of Haulbowline in Cork, at Portland, and at Walmer in Kent. Four sisters accompanied the hospital ship on the punitive expedition against the West African kingdom of Benin in 1897 and, with the medical officers and sick berth staff, had to deal with over 1000 cases of malarial fever. At the beginning of the twentieth century sisters were also serving in Hong Kong, Gibraltar and at various naval establishments in the United Kingdom.

In 1902 Queen Alexandra indicated her 'great wish . . . to have the Navy Nursing Department under her special charge . . . and that it . . . bear her name.' Its title thus became Queen Alexandra's Royal Naval Nursing Service (QARNNS) and for many years Queen Alexandra personally signed the paper confirming each sister found suitable for appointment in the service.

The bestowal of royal patronage entailed a change in uniform. The earlier grey serge gown had been replaced by the more appropriate navy blue, and now scarlet cuffs were added. The Geneva cross was moved from the right arm to form part of the distinctive insignia worn on the new tippet. The original frilled cap, tied under the chin, gave way to a handkerchief-style 'veil' as the head-dress is known still. A scarlet-hooded navy blue serge cloak with a navy blue straw bonnet was worn outdoors. The uniform has changed little since except for fluctuations in skirt length in line with fashion and the addition of a new tricorn outdoor hat.

Periodically the uniform has been adapted to meet the needs of active service, the most recent example being during the Falklands War when trousers and pullovers were worn.

Naval nursing in wartime

At the outbreak of the First World War in 1914 there were 69 sisters in the service. This number was quickly augmented by the addition of 200 sisters from the reserve formed in 1910 by volunteer nurses from civilian hospitals. During the war nursing sisters and members of the Voluntary Aid Detachment (VAD) served in home naval hospitals at Portsmouth, Plymouth, Chatham, Deal, Shotley and Portland, and abroad in Malta, Hong Kong and Gibraltar. On the hospital ships, to which only QARNNS sisters were appointed, they frequently, as in the case of the ships anchored off the Gallipoli Peninsula, worked in conditions of great danger. After the armistice hospital ships were still required to transfer home former prisoners of war from Europe and also to care for the German sick and wounded from the surrendered battle fleet at Scapa Flow. Nine sisters were killed during the hostilities and sixteen Royal Red Cross medals were awarded.

During the interwar years the number of nurses in the service gradually increased to 85. This number rose to 193 in 1939, when, as in 1914, the service was rapidly increased by reserve sisters and VADs to meet the expanding needs of a nation at war and finally reached approximately 1300. By the end of the war they were employed in the existing naval hospitals, the six auxiliary hospitals and in the many sick quarters provided wherever the members of the Women's Royal Naval Service were training and serving, at home and abroad, from Grimsby to Hong Kong and from the Isle of Man to Trincomalee. Sisters were present during the bombardment of Malta and at the capture of Hong Kong in 1941 by the Japanese, by whom they were interned for the remainder of the war. They served at the base hospital at Alexandria which initially took the majority of the casualties from the Eighth Army's offensive in Libya in 1942, and were on board HMHS *Oxfordshire* when it embarked the wounded from Tunisia while fighting was still in progress. For a short time, in Australia, sisters took to the air, acting as flight nurses during the evacuation of casualties from the Admiralty Islands to Sydney.

The work of hospital ships was mainly confined to the Far East, where they were used for the repatriation of prisoners of war from the Philippines to Canada via Pearl Harbor and Hong Kong. In unusual, difficult and sometimes dangerous conditions, despite curtailed training periods, shortages of equipment and the fact that the regular sisters, familiar with naval routine, were scattered worldwide, naval sisters maintained a high level of professional competence. Twelve

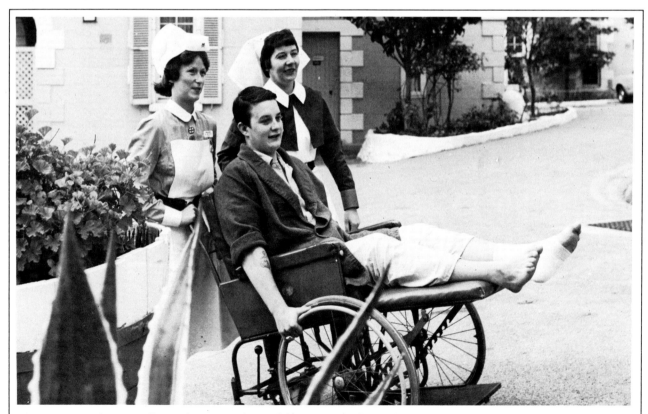

A naval nursing officer and a nurse with one of their patients at the Royal Naval Hospital, Gibraltar, in the 1960s.

members of QARNNS died on active service and over 100 decorations were awarded.

In 1949, on the formation of the medical branch of the Women's Royal Naval Service, WRNS sick berth attendants were trained and worked alongside the male branch, established in 1884. VADs still remaining in the navy were given the option of retaining their separate identity or joining the newly formed WRNS branch, which continued until 1960 when it was replaced, along with the remaining VADs, by new QARNNS ratings. QARNNS therefore became a two-tier service: sisters, selected from applicants who were state registered nurses, and nurses, under training for state registration or state enrolment. Nursing ratings now join the navy at HMS *Raleigh* and continue professional training at the Portsmouth District and Royal Naval School of Nursing, following the curriculum laid down by the General Nursing Council.

A non-nursing section, known as the Clerical and Quarters Category, was introduced in 1974, its purpose being to provide officers and ratings whose task is to manage QARNNS quarters, administration and welfare in Royal Naval hospitals at home and abroad.

In 1977 QARNNS personnel became subject to naval discipline and commissions were granted to nursing officers. From April 1982 it became a unified service and for the first time men were given the opportunity to join. Medical technicians and assistants, whose duties had evolved from those of the original sick berth attendants of 1884, could, with the necessary qualifications, transfer from their branches to the Royal Navy. Additionally, men qualified as state registered nurses became eligible to apply for short service commissions. The all-female naval nursing service was just two years short of its century.

QARNNS, like any other branch of the services, had to react swiftly to the crisis over the Falkland Islands. The SS *Uganda* served as the hospital ship for the three services during the conflict in 1982. Its complement consisted of 15 QARNNS female officers, 31 female ratings (at this time the integration of men into the service had not been effected), 23 medical assistants and technicians, and 10 medical officers. SS *Uganda* was the first British hospital ship since HMHS *Maine*, which saw action in the Korean War, and it was also the first time since that war that female nurses had served at sea.

At very short notice and with only three days of intensive training, concentrating on burns, gunshot wounds and trauma, the team flew to Gibraltar where they boarded *Uganda* for the voyage south. As they went, the hospital was unpacked from its crates and public rooms were transformed to accommodate an operating theatre, a pathology laboratory, wards, and burns and intensive care units. During the two months the ship spent in the war zone its medical team treated 730 casualties, including 150 Argentine prisoners. More than 500 operations were performed despite adverse weather conditions. Many of the wounds and burns were horrific, and not commonly seen in peacetime

hospitals. Moreover, the wounded could and did arrive at an alarmingly swift rate. In such circumstances nursing resources were strained to their maximum but all members of QARNNS responded with initiative, courage and resolution.

Today QARNNS personnel continue their responsibility for the health and fitness of all who belong to the Royal Navy, the Royal Marines and the Women's Royal Naval Service at sick bays and medical centres at naval establishments throughout the country and abroad in such places as Lisbon and Gibraltar. The Royal Naval hospitals at Haslar and Stonehouse are still the focal points of naval medicine, where dockyard employees and civilians from the local areas also receive treatment. In fact, the professional and personal qualities of QARNNS have established the service as part of the traditions and history of the Royal Navy, while it also continues to enjoy the benefits of the progress of modern medicine.

Nursing in the RAF

On 1 April 1918 the Royal Air Force was formed from the union of the Royal Flying Corps and the Royal Naval Air Service. Nursing care of the sick and wounded had, until this time, been in the hands of the army and naval nursing services. Because RAF stations were widely scattered, it soon became obvious that there was a requirement for a nursing service within easy reach of the airfields and training camps. This nursing service was formed in June 1918, with a strength of 42 nurses.

In June 1923 King George V gave his assent for the RAF nursing service to be known as Princess Mary's Royal Air Force Nursing Service (PMRAFNS). However, it was not until Oct. 1950, following the integration of the PMRAFNS with the RAF, that King George VI gave his approval for the appointment of their patron, the Princess Royal (Princess Mary), as Air Chief Commandant PMRAFNS.

During her lifetime the Princess Royal was closely associated with the growth and development of the service, and gave her name to its oldest hospital at Halton and its newest one at Akrotiri in Cyprus. She paid frequent visits to the hospitals at home and abroad, and did much to raise the morale of the servicemen and women. In 1966, after the Princess Royal's death in the previous year, Princess Alexandra was appointed her successor.

Miss Jolly, of Guy's Hospital, was the first matron-in-chief, but served only a few months because of ill-health. Her place was taken by Joanna Cruikshank, who was matron-in-chief for 12 years and the true founder of PMRAFNS. She was a dynamic personality, possessing great drive and energy, encouraging the sisters through the difficult years of personal hardships they had to endure at the beginning. Their salary was £60 a year, and they worked under very poor conditions, often in old hutted buildings

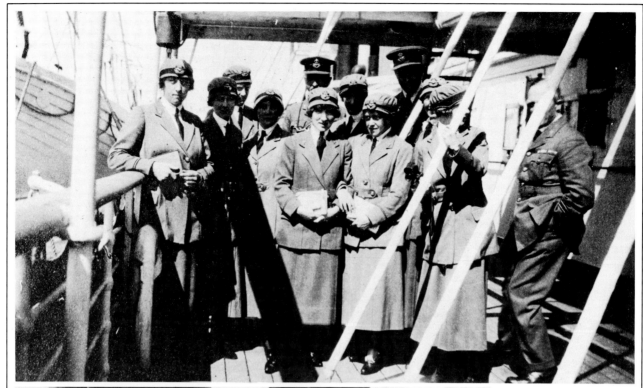

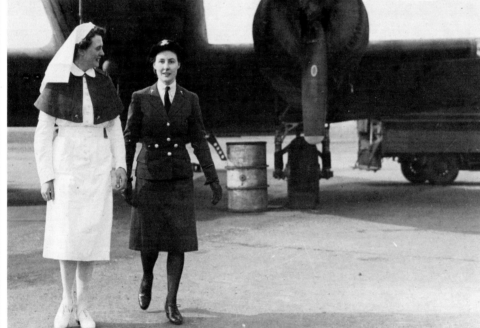

Above *Members of PMRAFNS on board ship on their way to take up duties in Baghdad, Iraq, in the 1920s.*
Left *PMRAFNS sisters on an airfield in Britain in 1944 wearing the indoor uniform of white with a blue cape and the outdoor uniform consisting of a tunic and skirt in air force blue.*

with no running water. One of the pioneers recalled patients pulling wool from their dressings to plug holes in the walls of their huts and stop the draughts. At one hospital the sisters even had to work by the light of hurricane lamps, walking knee-deep in mud from one hut to another during the cold winter months. Snow had to be melted to provide water for tea and dressings, and four sisters had to sleep on the floor of an operating room for several weeks until some kind local people offered them accommodation in their homes. Since

those early pioneer days, the PMS, as they are affectionately known throughout the RAF, have certainly lived up to the motto of the RAF medical services – *Nec Aspera Terrent* ('Nothing will deter us').

In May 1923 the first ten sisters to go overseas were posted to hospitals in Baghdad and Basrah. They travelled by sea accompanied by over 1000 officers and men of the RAF on the liner *Braemar Castle*, the first troopship hired exclusively for the RAF.

In 1927 the new hospital at RAF Halton was opened by the Princess Royal. It was later to become famous for its burns and plastic surgery unit, and since 1957 the renal unit, with mobile teams on 24-hour standby, has always been ready for duty anywhere in the United Kingdom or abroad.

The Second World War and after

During the early years of the Second World War there was no lack of volunteers for nursing with the armed forces. PMRAFNS nursing sisters, RAF and WRAF nursing attendants, aided by VADs, with nursing sisters of the British Red Cross Society, and nursing members of the Canadian forces, cared for the sick and wounded in RAF hospitals. These nursing service personnel also worked in the sick quarters, the large training wings, recruiting centres and schools of technical training. With the increased numbers of women in the RAF, nursing sisters were appointed as welfare nursing officers to assist medical officers in the care of the female element of the service.

The nursing sisters served with their medical colleagues in every combat area in which the RAF was engaged. There were additional general hospitals and sick quarters in the United Kingdom and overseas in Iraq, Palestine, Libya, Egypt, Iceland, West Africa, India and the Bahamas. Mobile field hospitals were set up in various towns in tented accommodation and in commandeered buildings in Burma, Singapore, the Western Desert, Italy, France, the Netherlands, Algeria, on the North African coast, and in Sicily and Sardinia.

In 1941, in order to bring the nursing sisters in line with other servicewomen, they were granted emergency wartime commissions. They wore officers' rank markings on their uniform, but were still addressed by their professional titles. Their salaries remained in accordance with civilian nurses' scales. By the beginning of 1943, 1125 nursing sisters staffed the 32 RAF hospitals functioning at that time. In addition to these hospitals, there were 71 station sick quarters and 47 stations with welfare sisters. In Marcy 1943 the PMRAFNS were granted emergency commissions in the Women's Defence Forces for the duration of the war and began work in the mobile field hospitals. These hospitals moved around in the field of battle, but were usually situated near airfields for the convenience of aeromedical evacuation. Transport aircraft were converted into air ambulances and patients carried to safety as soon as they were fit to travel.

At critical times during the fighting in the Western Desert PMRAFNS personnel manning the mobile field hospitals moved forward with the Allied forces. They arrived on the beaches at Salerno, Italy, in tank landing craft while under enemy fire. Plans for the invasion of Europe found them concerned in the treatment of men wounded in seaborne landings and in the evacuation of casualties to hospitals in Britain. Many sisters landed on the Continent within seven days of the initial D-Day landings, and travelled with the mobile field hospitals through France and Belgium to Germany. Throughout these operations they also served on troopships which were under RAF control. However, in spite of their being torpedoed and being forced to spend a day or two in open boats, there was not a single major casualty amongst the ranks of the PMRAFNS.

Nurse training began in the RAF in 1951 when the General Nursing Council approved four major RAF Hospitals as nurse training schools for RAF and WRAF personnel. When the non-commissioned element of the PMRAFNS was formed in April 1963, suitably qualified candidates were transferred from the WRAF for nurse training. Thereafter, student nurses were recruited directly into the non-commissioned elements of the PMRAFNS. Student nurse training for state registration was discontinued in 1977. However, enrolled nurse (general) training had started in 1967, and was still being carried out in the 1980s in the two remaining nurse training schools, at Princess Alexandra's Hospital, Wroughton, and at RAF Hospital Ely.

During the period 1968–80 there was a gradual reduction in the overall establishment of the RAF. Withdrawal of British armed forces from the Middle and Far East brought with it the shutting down of a number of overseas hospitals, and the reduced size of the RAF necessitated the closure of some of the smaller hospitals in the United Kingdom. Today, members of the PMRAFNS serve at RAF medical centres at home and overseas, and at the three RAF hospitals in the United Kingdom – Ely, Halton and Wroughton – and overseas in Cyprus and Germany. Prior to 1980, the PMRAFNS had its own rank structure, and was restricted to female nursing officers and nurses, but on 1 April 1980, when the RAF's unified nursing service was inaugurated, PMRAFNS became a complete nursing service. All male registered nurses and enrolled nurses were now members of the PMRAFNS, resulting in equal opportunities for promotion to top level posts for commissioned officers and for airmen and airwomen to the rank of warrant officer.

Aeromedical evacuation is an integral part of the PMRAFNS. The first flight on record was in 1918 in a converted DH6 at Helwan in Egypt. The patient was loaded on a stretcher into a cut-out section of the fuselage and the aperture covered with canvas. Later, during operations in Somaliland in 1919, the RAF moved three patients 175 miles on stretchers fixed on to the fuselage of a DH9. In 1925 the first air ambulance service in the United Kingdom was established at RAF Halton. In 1933 the RAF carried 359 patients in Vickers Vernons and Vickers Victorias, and the aeromedical service began to develop, chiefly overseas in Iraq. The largest number of casualties evacuated by air in one year was recorded as 300,000 in 1944 from western Europe, the Mediterranean and the Far East. The tiny Vickers Vernons have long since been replaced by the VC10 and Hercules aircraft of today's RAF. Casualty experiences gained in Korea, Burma, Malaya, Aden and Cyprus proved invaluable during the Falklands conflict in 1982.

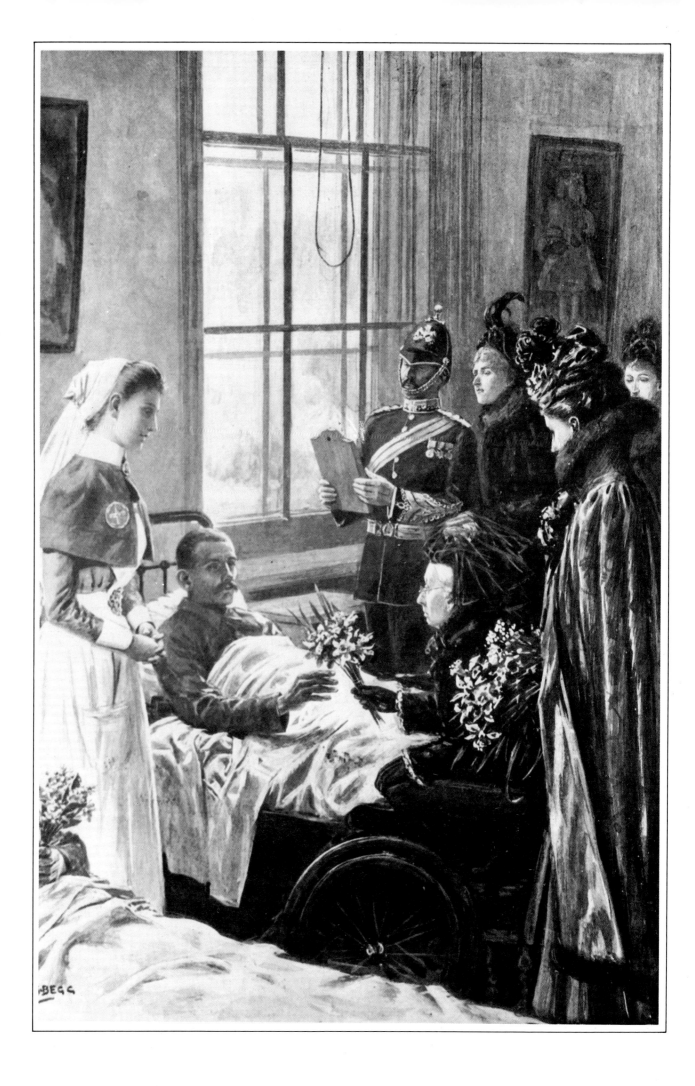

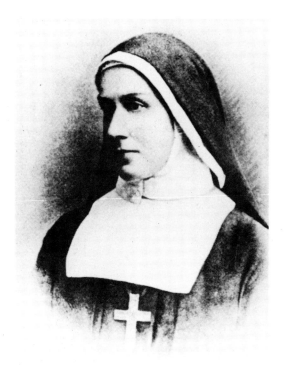

Nursing in the Boer War and South Africa

The outbreak of war

When the British government's dispute with the Boers culminated on 11 Oct. 1899 in an ultimatum, few anticipated a serious or long-drawn out campaign. So far as the British public was concerned, South Africa was a land as remote as the moon, a place peopled by savages, wild beasts and intransigent and backward Boer farmers. It was generally felt that the queen's 'dear' soldiers would speedily trounce the presumptuous Afrikaners.

To everyone's surprise the Boers, having demanded that British troops in, or on their way to, South Africa should be withdrawn, invaded Natal where the first engagement took place. The artillery of the Boers was superb and their tactics excellent, but the British regulars, numbering around 4000, were seasoned soldiers, and both sides could claim successes. Suddenly what was happening was no longer an incident to be dismissed, but had the makings of a real war.

Top *Sister Henrietta Stockdale, a member of an Anglican order of nuns, who did so much to establish nursing on a proper basis in South Africa.*
Opposite *Queen Victoria presents a bunch of flowers to a soldier while visiting the wounded at the Royal Herbert Hospital, Woolwich, during the Boer War of 1899–1902.*

At the outset of the war the Army Nursing Service had about 100 members, comprising a lady superintendent, 19 superintendents and 68 nurses. It was obvious that more nurses would be required to look after the needs of the biggest army Britain had ever sent abroad. To process and administer all offers of voluntary help, the National Aid Society, the St John Ambulance Association and the Army Nursing Service Reserve formed themselves into the Central Red Cross Committee. They delegated to the Army Nursing Service Reserve (ANSR) the task of sorting out the offers from nurses anxious to help. Eventually about 1800 nursing sisters served in South Africa, many of them recruited through the ANSR, with contingents from Canada, Australia, New Zealand and a group selected by the Princess of Wales (later Queen Alexandra).

Twenty-two general hospitals were opened in South Africa, each staffed with a complement of over 20 nurses. Four sisters were attached to each base hospital on the lines of communication, and two to each of the seven modern and well-found hospital trains. Although sisters did not officially serve with the field hospitals set up in tents and moved together with the army, a number of nurses found their way to the field hospitals.

Conditions in the base hospitals were better than those found by Florence Nightingale and her nurses at Scutari and, though there was still enough red tape to strangle all initiative, the personnel and troops were better housed and fed, besides receiving additional supplies sent in Red Cross parcels.

The British Red Cross had early made contingency plans. Colonel J. S. Young was appointed chief commissioner, and was instructed to bring together the various societies formed in South Africa for helping the sick and wounded. He reached South Africa on 14 Nov., at almost the same time as the army commander, Sir Redvers Buller.

On arriving at Cape Town Colonel Young reported to the military authorities to offer the assistance of the Red Cross, and he arranged with the Good Hope Red Cross Society and the local St John Ambulance Association that they should all work together as a team. He sent home for two assistant commissioners, who were immediately posted to Cape Town to join him.

Colonel Young had a difficult task. He had to organize voluntary aid throughout the Cape Colony and Natal, and send help with each of the three relieving columns. He visited hospital trains and also the hospital at Wynberg, where he made a special point of seeing the Boer prisoners.

Committees of ladies anxious to help were speedily formed. Each week the hospitals received a consignment of the latest London daily and illustrated papers, which were sorted and packed and distributed weekly by committee members. It was they who supervised the supply of warm clothing to invalids leaving Cape Town for England. Their most important work, however, was to meet the hospital trains when they arrived filled with casualties, handing out cold drinks, fruit, milk, eggs, and other comforts. Moreover, each train, as it left Cape Town for the front, was given a supply of hospital kits to be distributed to the sick and wounded as soon as they were entrained. The kits were put in linen bags stamped in red letters 'The Gift of the Good Hope and British Red Cross Societies', and each bag contained pyjamas, slippers, a towel, a flannel shirt, a sponge bag and sponge, a pair of socks, a tooth brush, one cake of soap and a hairbrush. The wounded, who came to the trains straight from the battlefield, were delighted with their 'lucky bags' as they called them.

One of the hospital trains, the *Princess Christian*, had been the brainchild of one of Queen Victoria's daughters, and was very popular with the wounded, being comfortable and well equipped. The first carriage was divided into three compartments, one for linen and other stores, one for two nurses, and one for two invalid officers. The second consisted of rooms for two medical officers, a dining-room and a dispensary, while numbers three, four, five and six were each constructed to carry eighteen invalids and four hospital orderlies. The kitchen and pantry accommodation for two cooks was in the seventh coach, each carriage being provided with a stove, lavatory and closet. The *Princess Christian* could carry 97 passengers. On its arrival at the Cape in 1899 it was the object of much interest.

On 8 Jan. 1900 the hospital ship *Princess of Wales* arrived in Cape Town. She had originally been a yachting cruiser called the *Midnight Sun*, when she was found by a Major

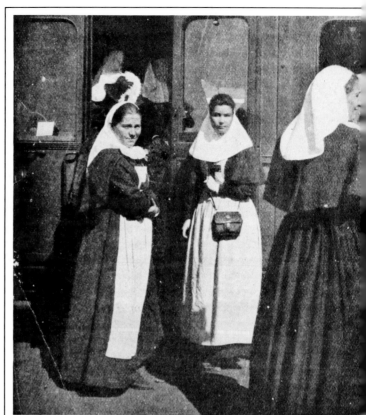

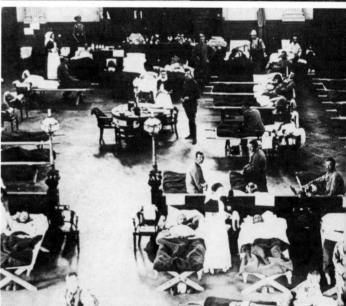

Top *Russian nurses with the Boer forces in the western Transvaal in 1900. Many European countries sympathized with the Boers in their struggle with the British.*
Above *The British army hospital in the Raadzaal, Bloemfontein, in 1900. Makeshift arrangements were frequently necessary to deal with the high casualty rate.*
Opposite, above *A tented British hospital in the grounds of the Ramblers' Club, Bloemfontein. From the* Illustrated London News, *9 June 1900.*
Opposite, below *The hospital for British officers at Wynberg, Cape Province. The patients appear to be well on the way to recovery.*

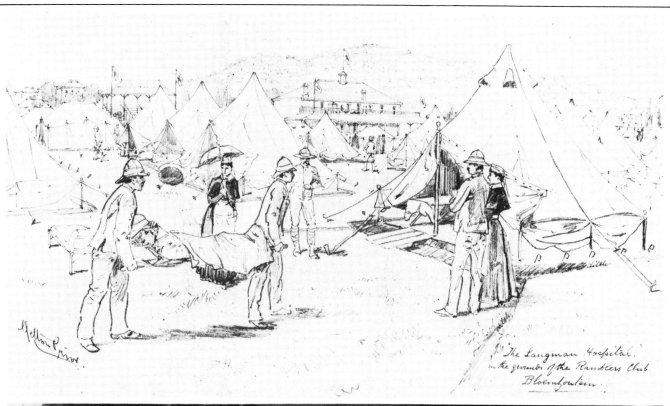

"The Langman Hospital" in the grounds of the Ramblers Club. Bloemfontein.

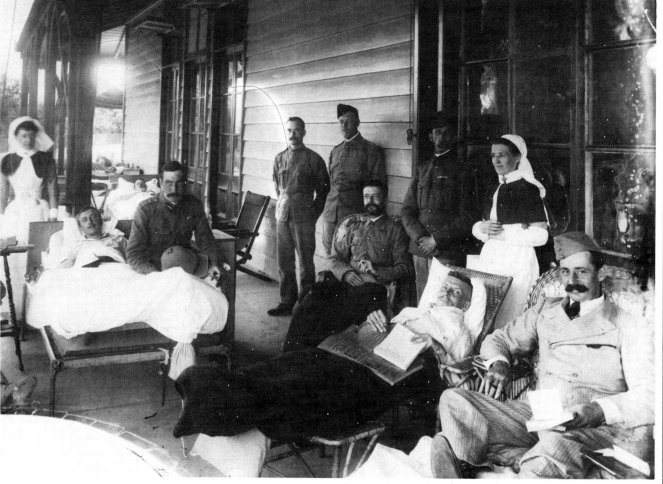

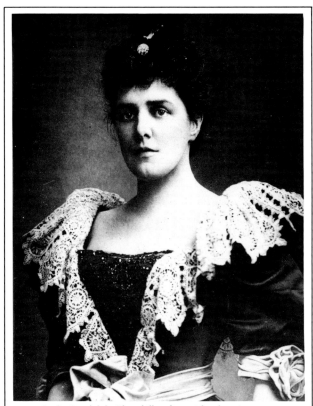

Lady Randolph Churchill, who, with other American women, helped to equip a hospital ship for service in South Africa.

Macpherson, to whom had fallen the unenviable task of purchasing suitable vessels at a time when all available shipping was required to transport troops. However, the conversion was finally accomplished to the satisfaction of the sponsors. The ship carried three surgeons, three nursing sisters, 23 orderlies of the Royal Army Medical Corps, and 23 men of the St John Ambulance Brigade. The *Princess of Wales* was to make three voyages between England and Cape Town, also carrying patients between Cape Town and East London.

Besides this ship, another, the *Maine*, was fitted out and run by a committee of American ladies in London, under the presidency of Lady Randolph Churchill, both of whose sons, Winston and Jack, were soldiering in South Africa. The idea of chartering a hospital ship had originated with another American woman, a Mrs Blow, who had spent some years in South Africa. The vessel was provided by Bernard N. Baker, president of the Atlantic Transport Company. After a widely publicized launching ceremony, the Duke of Connaught presented the *Maine* with a Union Jack from Queen Victoria.

The Sunday before the ship sailed for South Africa, the public were allowed aboard and much interest was shown, particularly by the women visitors, in Lady Randolph's own quarters, which 'resembled a lady's boudoir, rich in the luxuries of silken hangings and cushions'. To match her elegant quarters, Winston's mother had designed for herself

an eye-catching uniform consisting of a trim white jacket and skirt, embroidered blouse and 'matronish' starched white cap.

Much attention, too, had been given to the design of the uniform worn by the nurses sent out to South Africa. These were specially adapted to the hot climate and to coping with sand and mud. The grey uniform dress reached just above the ankle – a startling innovation! The sisters were also issued with straw boaters trimmed with a bright red ribbon, and a white parasol lined with scarlet.

Early nursing in South Africa

The first hospital in South Africa had been established by Jan van Riebeeck when in 1652, after 104 days at sea, three vessels of the Dutch East India Company cast anchor at the foot of Table Mountain. Van Riebeeck's instructions were to build a fort and erect a hospital within its precincts. Its functions were to accommodate the sick from passing ships. Though van Riebeeck had also been given instructions to appoint official midwives to the new trading station, the sick in the hospital were always attended by humble orderlies in the service of the company.

It was to be a long time before institutional nursing came to South Africa. It was not, as in Europe, a charitable or intellectual occupation, and it was not until the arrival of settlers from Britain in 1820 that the pattern of civilian nursing can be said to have taken root. Their coming had a profound effect on the development of medical and military matters in the eastern Cape, and subsequently in the whole of the Cape region. As towns and villages arose, the settlers demanded hospitals and schools, demands ignored by a colonial government which would later deeply regret its neglect of their wishes.

In attendance on the sick in military depots were military orderlies, supervised by a sergeant supposed to be experienced in medical matters. During the Kaffir Wars the wives of these men shared in the nursing work, so that an efficient cadre of men and women with knowledge of hospital matters was formed in the area. Thus, when civilian hospitals were finally established, a relatively experienced nursing force was available.

A series of small general hospitals were opened in the mid-1850s, and in 1874 the first nurses trained in the Nightingale pattern were sent out to South Africa. In this same year the first Anglican sisters arrived, some of whom had been trained under the Anglican sisterhood in London. The advent of the nurses of the Anglican sisterhood was ultimately to lead to the world's first statutory registration, that of the nurses of the Cape, in 1891.

The Order of St Thomas the Martyr sent Sister Emma, with five associates, to found an Anglican nursing and teaching order at Bloemfontein in the Orange Free State. One of these five associates was the famous Henrietta

Stockdale, the pioneer of trained nursing. Sister Stockdale was to become known, not only for service in the siege of Kimberley, but also because, together with three other sisters, she volunteered to reorganize the department of the lepers who had been isolated on Robben Island, off Cape Town. The sisters stayed long enough to institute a proper nursing service for the unfortunate lepers, and to find suitable attendants to care for them.

Sister Henrietta, as sister in charge of the Carnavon Hospital, Kimberley, had started a training school there. At the Somerset Hospital, Cape Town, the oldest hospital in South Africa, the training of nurses was begun in 1886 by Sister Mary Agatha of the All Saints Sisterhood. Other schools were established at the Albany General Hospital, Grahamstown, the Provincial Hospital, Port Elizabeth, and Grey's Hospital, Pietermaritzburg. The vast Johannesburg hospital, which began as a series of tents, was at first staffed by Roman Catholic sisters, but in 1895 some qualified lay nurses were selected in England.

Effects of the war

The South African War was to have a tremendous impact on the nurses. At first they had to care only for the wounded in their neat, clean, hygienic hospitals well away from the front, but as the tides of war began to wash over the whole country, many of the nurses found themselves closer to the front lines than ever before, living in tents and being suddenly overwhelmed by casualties and by two new and terrible enemies – enteric and typhoid.

The British Unionist MP, William Burdett Coutts, husband of the great philanthropist, Angela Burdett Coutts, described in *The Times*, as Russell had done before him in the Crimea, what he saw in Bloemfontein:

> 'Hundreds of men to my knowledge were lying in the worst stages of typhoid, with only a blanket and a thin waterproof sheet (not even the latter for many of them) between their aching bodies and the hard ground; with no milk and hardly any medicines, without beds, stretcher or mattresses, without linen of any kind. . . .'

Why was there a typhoid epidemic? Because the men, who had not been warned, stopped to drink water whenever and wherever they found it. They had drunk deep of the water of the Modder River at Paardeberg, polluted by Cronje's camp.

Much of the blame for the number of deaths was due to the failure of one single-track railway line, lacking the rolling stock to supply all the needs of the army. There were

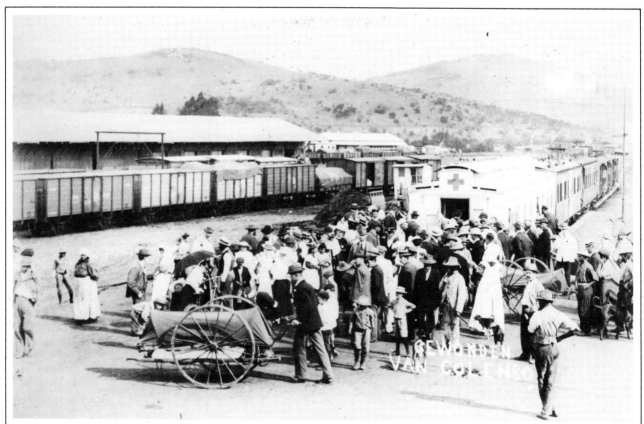

Wounded men being disembarked from a hospital train after the Battle of Colenso in Dec. 1899 in which British forces suffered heavy losses.

volunteer hospitals at Bloemfontein staffed by civilian doctors, including Conan Doyle. There was also a Boer government hospital, the Volks Hospital, whose staff did all they could to help the wounded and sick British soldiers, but they, too, were utterly dependent on that single-track railway line.

Nurses caught up in the sieges of Kimberley, Ladysmith and Mafeking worked to exhaustion. Sister Henrietta in her hospital in Kimberley wrote:

> 'At Christmas there was a great strain upon all our resources. Every moment of my time was spent trying to spin out our wretched scraps of horse-flesh, and our few ounces of milk in our own household.'

On 15 Feb. 1900, the army flooded into Kimberley, and Sister Henrietta again recorded her experiences. She wrote that she and her nurses worked 'through the whole day, standing in the furiously hot little operating room, or dressing ghastly wounds, almost standing on our heads for the men were all on the floor. Indeed the heat is almost indescribable. . . .'

Yet, regardless of epidemics, mosquitoes, flies, snakes,

fierce ants, dust storms, rainstorms and a shortage of almost everything, the nurses followed the Nightingale example. This was in spite of the principal medical officer, Surgeon-General Wilson, who, when being told of the urgent need for more nurses, 'was not very responsive or sympathetic' to the idea of women nurses.

During the siege of Ladysmith, Mother Marie-des-Anges left her comfortable convent to the British soldiers and the Boers and, accompanied by her small community of nurses, drove out to Intombi Spruit, four miles southeast of Ladysmith, to the field hospital, whose tents were crammed with sick and wounded. The nuns worked valiantly among them until they too, one by one, fell victim to dysentery or enteric fever.

Nursing care in the field was generally provided by the orderlies, but in some battles the wives of British soldiers came to the help of the wounded. Two of them received awards. Marion Smith for the 'good service she rendered after the Bronthorstspruit affair', was given a silver medal and a Diploma of the Order of St John of Jerusalem. Sister Louise and a Mrs Maistre were each awarded the Royal Red Cross in recognition of their sterling work with typhoid patients.

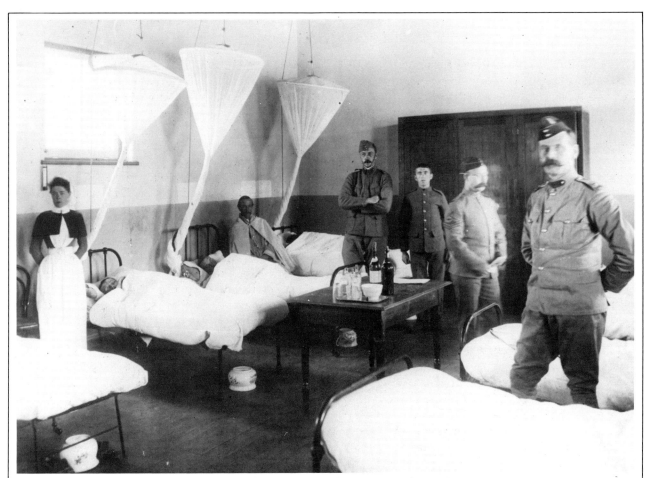

A ward in a British military hospital in South Africa. Conditions had vastly improved since the Crimean War, but the nursing staff had to contend with typhoid and other diseases as well as wounds and often worked in difficult and dangerous conditions.

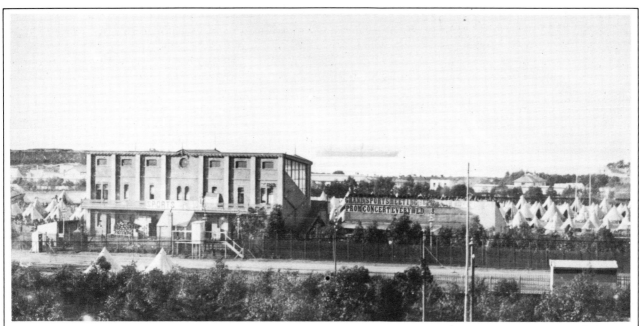

A camp for Boer prisoners at Cape Town, c.1900. Despite the discomforts of their tented accommodation they fared much better than their womenfolk in the concentration camps.

The concentration camps

Sombre as was the picture of the sick and wounded casualties on both sides, there was an even darker aspect to the Boer War – a grievance that has affected relations between the British and the Afrikaners to this day. This was the establishment of the concentration camps. The expression was taken from the Spanish word *reconcentrado*, used in connection with the camps set up by the Spanish to deal with guerrillas after the Cuban rebellion of 1895.

It is probable that little would have been heard of the thousands of Afrikaner women and children herded into camps if a dumpy, middle-aged spinster with a genius for winkling out unpalatable truths had not toured what were known as the 'burgher refugee camps'. What Emily Hobhouse saw on this tour so appalled her that she determined that the whole world should hear what supposedly decent Englishmen had done to the population of the country they had overrun by force of arms.

Emily Hobhouse had influential Liberal connections. Indeed, it was through these that she had met Lord Milner who had naïvely arranged for her to visit the refugee camps. On her return to Britain she lost no time in mounting her crusade and of informing the world of what was happening in South Africa. She spoke of 'the wholesale burning of farms . . . deportations . . . a burnt-out population brought in by hundreds of convoys . . . lack of food, clothes, medicines and even the barest necessities'. She also told of the famine and epidemics which raged through the camps.

It was not long before her story reached the press and it was obvious that her statements could not go unchallenged.

Accordingly, as a bold experiment, a 'ladies only commission' was formed to report on the true state of the concentration camps. The chairman, Mrs Millicent Fawcett, was an active Liberal Unionist, feminist and a leader of the women's suffrage movement. The five other members included Lady Knox, the wife of one of Lord Kitchener's generals, a nurse from Guy's Hospital, and two doctors who were already on duty in South Africa.

In July 1901 the commission journeyed up and down the countryside in one of the trains put at its disposal. In December it presented its findings in the shape of an official report. In their criticisms of the camp system, Millicent Fawcett and her group confirmed all that Emily Hobhouse had previously stated. Among their recommendations they urged that 40 trained nurses should be sent out to the camps without delay, that rations should be increased, that wood be provided for bedsteads, since internees had to sleep on the ground, that every camp should have the proper apparatus for sterilizing linen used by typhoid patients, and that a travelling inspector of camps should be appointed, as well as a number of camp matrons.

Mrs Fawcett's report was just and without any attempt to gloss over matters. It is interesting to note that though the commission had visited thirty-three *white* concentration camps, they had failed to visit a single camp for Africans, although there were many of these.

The final conclusions of the commission were scarifying. Muddle, red tape, bungling and lack of proper communications, they reported, had led to the deaths of 20,000 Europeans and 12,000 Africans and Coloured people. Their deaths were due in the main to epidemics, typhoid, dysentery, measles and malnutrition.

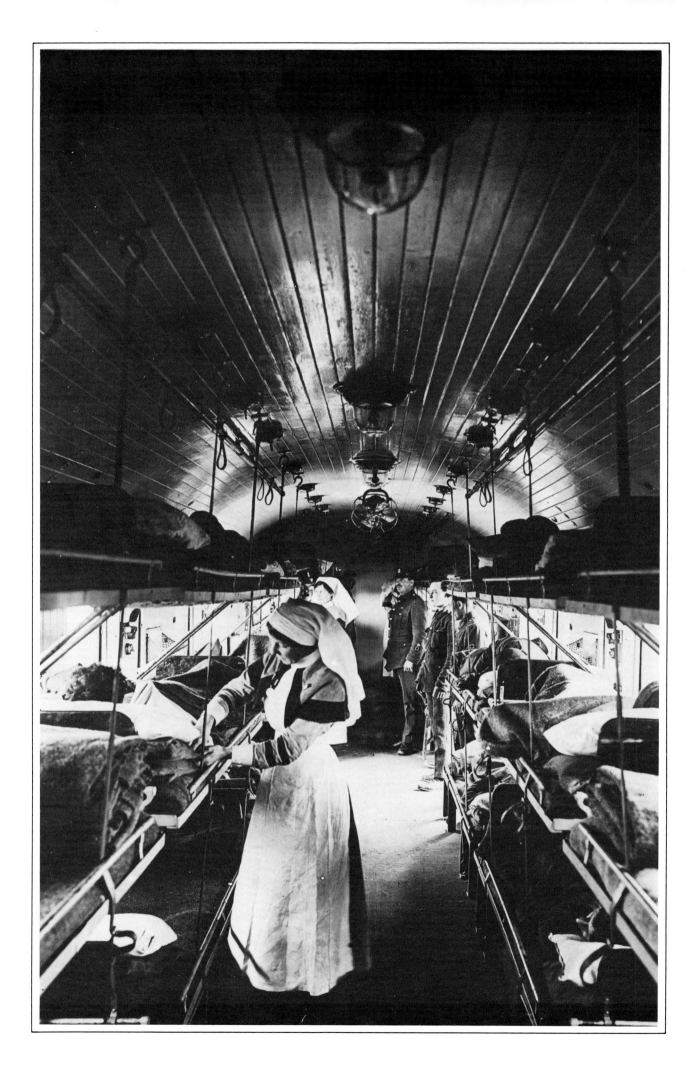

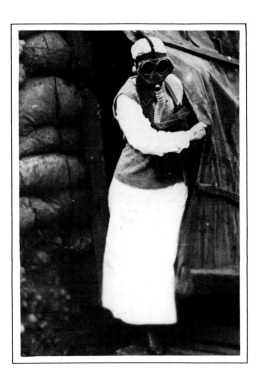

Nursing in the First World War

The VADs and others

As the British government's ultimatum to Germany expired on the evening of 4 Aug. 1914, the Foreign Secretary, Sir Edward Grey, watched the gas lights being dimmed in Whitehall, and said sadly, 'The lights are going out all over Europe, we shall not see them lit again in our lifetime.' This was a very different war from either the Crimean or the Boer War, for it meant the involvement of many countries and a tremendous upheaval in the nursing profession. The demand for nurses at home and on the various fronts was unprecedented. It had to be met by increased recruitment, by reducing the provision for the civilian sick, and by admitting large numbers of untrained or partially trained women to hospital work in Voluntary Aid Detachments.

The VAD scheme had come into being in Aug. 1909. It was organized by a joint committee of the Red Cross and the Order of St John of Jerusalem. When the war began there were approximately 80,000 members, and when it ended their numbers had increased to 120,000, of which there were 12,000 VAD nursing members working in military hospitals, while 60,000 members were employed in auxiliary hospitals. These were unpaid.

Top *An American nurse in a trench wearing a gas mask. The introduction of poison gas by the Germans in April 1915 added a new dimension to the horrors of modern warfare.*
Opposite *The interior of a ward on a British ambulance train near Doullens in northern France in April 1918.*

The uniform worn by the VADs comprised 11 items, including a dark blue rough serge overcoat with belt, 'Sister Dora' cap, and an apron with pockets with the red cross on the bib. The new VADs used to bleach the bright red crosses on their aprons so that they would look like the much-washed and faded crosses on the aprons worn by colleagues who had been working in hospitals since the beginning. They would also sprinkle themselves with carbolic or ether, which gave them the much-desired 'hospital' smell.

The VADs, who came in the main from the higher social classes, were not looked upon with any great favour by the trained nurses. Many of the new recruits passed overnight from the status of young society woman to that of adult in an ill-fitting uniform, working all hours in makeshift hospitals. There they tended men with terrible wounds, watching young soldiers affected by poison gas spewing out their lungs, laying out the dead, and caring desperately while their patients haemorrhaged to death on the operating table. Doctors, nurses and VADs were worked off their feet. They had no time to eat and no proper sleep, and even the most experienced medics were devastated by the ravages of some of the wounds they were trying to treat – all of them infected with gas gangrene.

A number of young women who were later to become famous recorded their impressions of the war. Among them was Lady Diana Duff-Cooper who, having tried, and failed, to get to France, opted to nurse at Guy's Hospital, where her beauty acted like a tonic on her patients. Vera Brittain, the writer, was also eager to serve her country, and her war diary, *Testament of Youth*, is a fascinating document which records her adventures at home and abroad as a nurse.

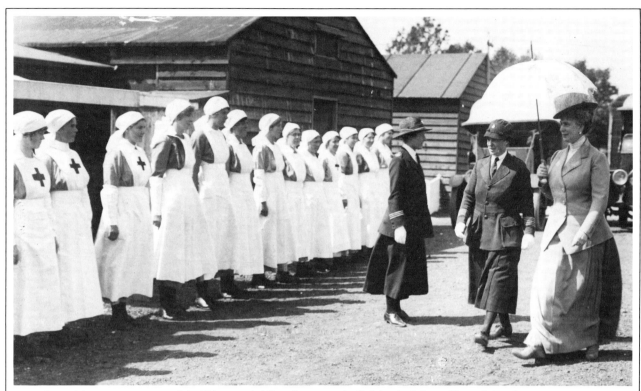

Queen Mary inspects nurses of the Voluntary Aid Detachments at the St John Ambulance Hospital, Etaples, France, in June 1917. The formation of VAD units had begun in 1909 and members were required to have certificates in first aid and home nursing.

Agatha Christie became a VAD as did Enid Bagnold who, despite protests from her family, went to work at a military hospital near London. Probably for the first time in her life she came face to face with the reality of pain. 'Six inches deep the gauze struck, crackling under the pull of the forceps, blood and pus leaping from the cavities.' She too was to keep a diary, which was a moving record of her experiences.

The landed gentry set a good example. It was patriotic to offer the family seat to the army as a divisional or corps headquarters. Most stately homes, however, were used as hospitals or convalescent homes. An appeal by the Duke of Sutherland to his peers resulted in instant offers of 250 country seats. Sadly, some of the most splendid castles in the realm were so deficient in basic amenities that they had to be rejected either as hospitals or convalescent homes.

The Nurses' Department was started in the early days of the war by Lady Gifford, who was then joined by Queen Amélie of Portugal. With the formation of the joint committee this department became unwieldy and obviously needed to be controlled by a professional. The woman chosen for this important post was Sarah Swift, who had recently resigned as matron of Guy's Hospital. The department provided the nursing staff for the auxiliary hospitals in the United Kingdom: 4730 were so employed; 762 trained nurses served in France and Belgium and 666 on other fronts, making a total of 6158, of which 365 subsequently joined the QAIMNS.

The authorities had made certain that this time they would not be caught napping as they had been in the Crimean War. There was a corps of army nurses. There were well-equipped hospitals in each command of Great Britain capable of caring for 7000 wounded. There were three hospital ships. There were cadres of trained personnel ready to set up field ambulances, casualty clearing stations and base hospitals. There was provision for a back-up organization of volunteers, for the army had realized that in the event of a European war its own resources would have to be supplemented by outside help.

The sick and wounded were to be found not only in France and Belgium, but also in Egypt and Mesopotamia, in Gallipoli, and in East Africa. In fact, wherever there were soldiers, there nurses went too. They had landed with the first contingent of the British Expeditionary Force in France in 1914. They wore close-fitting grey bonnets, tied with a bow under the chin, and under their travelling cloaks, ankle-length dresses covered with the short scarlet cape designed by Florence Nightingale. Some capes bore the red, yellow and blue ribbon of the South African campaign medal. All nurses wore the stiff, pink Alexandra rose at the back. Legend had it that the rose was thus placed to dig into the shoulder blades of any sister tempted to fall asleep on night duty.

In the First World War army and Red Cross nurses together numbered about 23,000, of whom 10,000 served overseas, many in base hospitals in the war zone or even

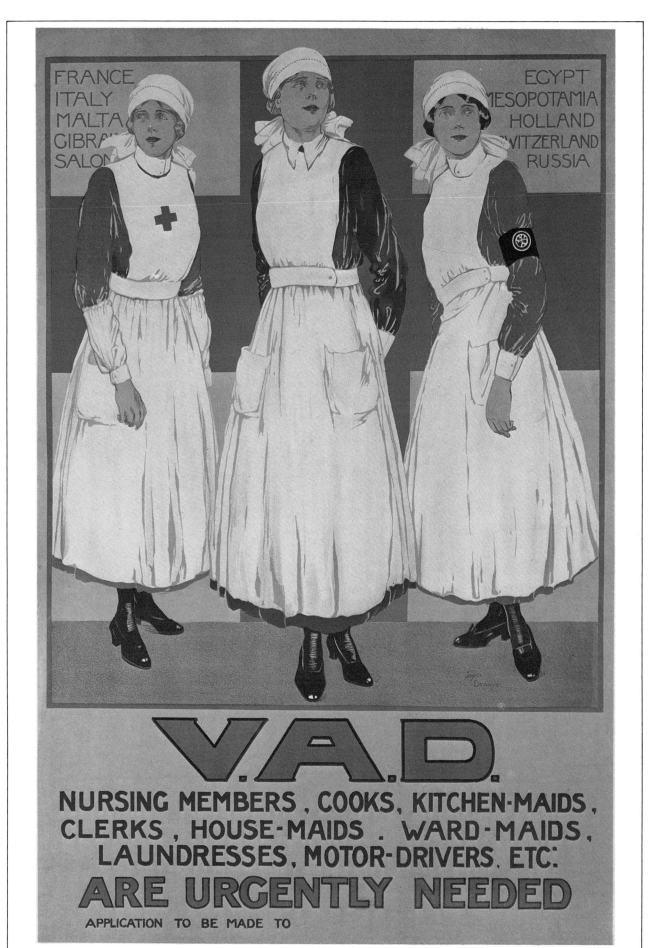

A First World War recruiting poster for the VAD. Despite the flood of volunteers at the beginning of the war, the mounting toll of casualties, both in France and in other theatres, led to a constant demand for more nurses.

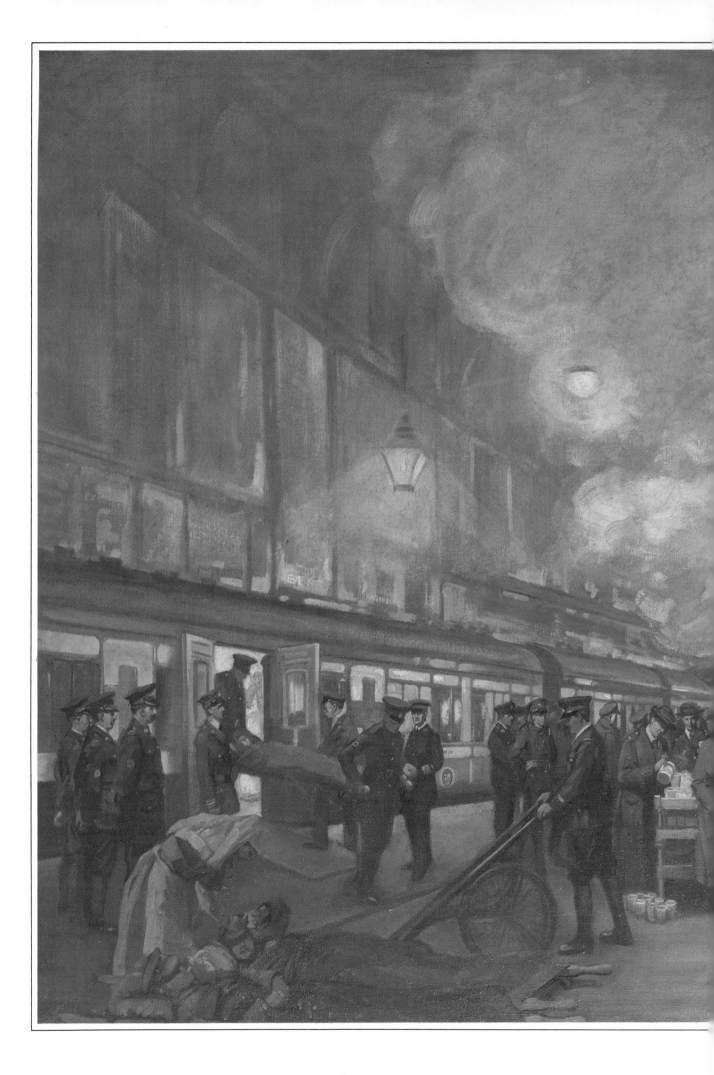

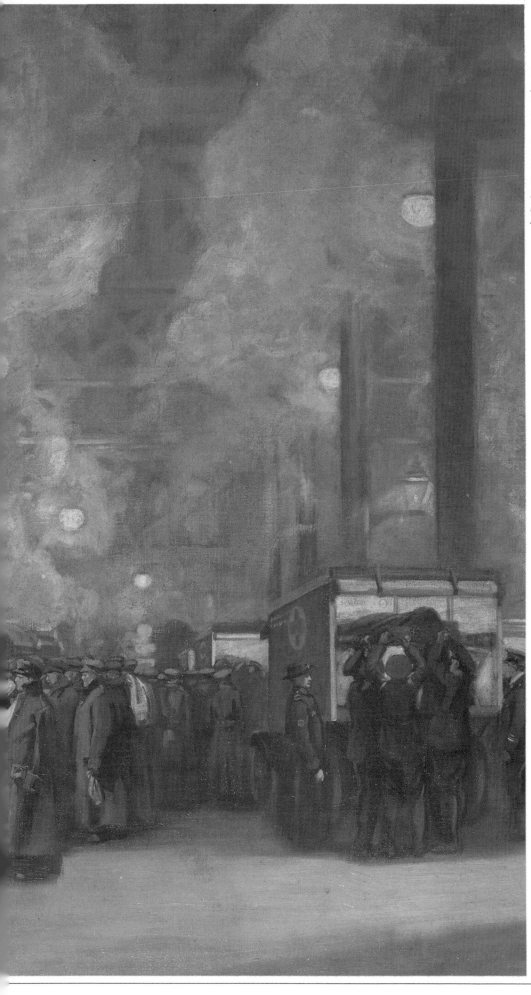

Soldiers wounded in the fighting in France being taken off a hospital train at Charing Cross station by members of the British Red Cross Society and the St John Ambulance Brigade. Such scenes were to become all too familiar as the war progressed. Painting by J. Hodgson Lobley, 1919.

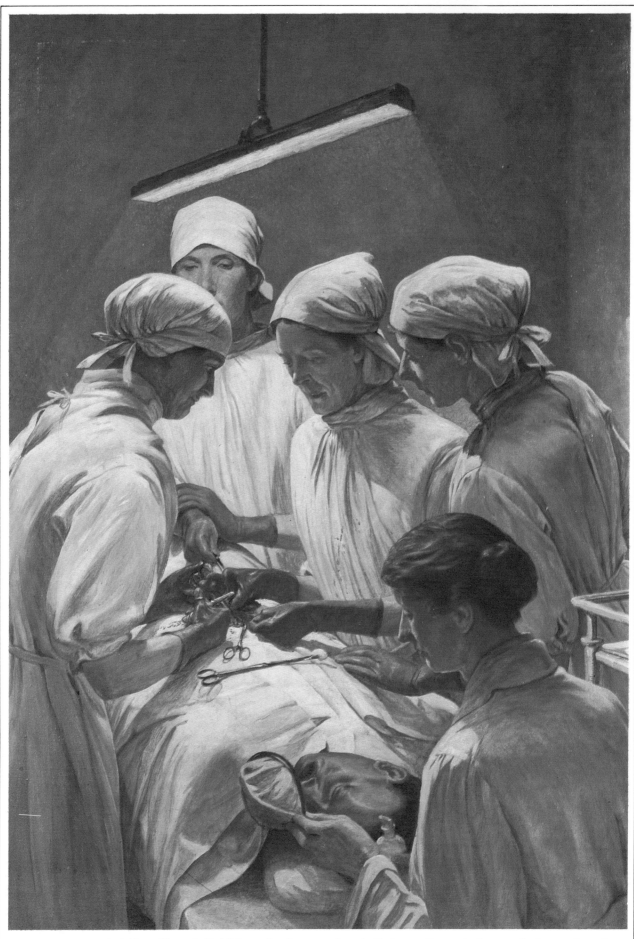

An operation at the Military Hospital, Endell Street, London, carried out by Dr Louisa Garrett Anderson and other members of the Women's Hospital Corps. Painting by Francis Dodd, 1920.

nearer the front. Hundreds of nurses from different countries died in the war, some of them drowned in hospital ships that were torpedoed.

The first army nursing service in Australia was formed in Sydney in 1898, and saw active service with the Australian troops in the South African War. In July 1902 the Australian Army Nursing Service was formally created.

The Canadian Military Nursing Service began with the employment of a few graduate nurses and religious sisters in the Saskatchewan Rebellion of 1884–5. In 1889, in General Military Orders it was stated that a definite nursing service was 'in contemplation', and four Canadian nurses went off to the Boer War. Two years later a nursing service was established as an integral part of the Canadian Army Medical Corps. It was reorganized in 1904, and in 1906 a Reserve Corps of 57 nursing sisters was formed. In 1919, in recognition of its war record, the service became the Royal Canadian Medical Corps.

The FANY

Within 24 hours of war being declared a unit of the First Aid Nursing Yeomanry (FANY), fresh from the hard training of their summer camp, was preparing for action. The corps was headed for Belgium and, with the paint still wet on their ambulance, the first unit left for Folkestone on 26 Oct. 1914. Among them were four trained nurses, a male ambulance driver and two male dressers.

On 29 Oct. the first FANY hospital, containing 100 beds, was opened in Calais. Housed in a convent school, it was in a thoroughly delapidated condition when taken over by the FANY. There was no equipment, and the first patients, mainly typhoid cases, were accommodated on straw or palliasses.

The history of the FANY makes colourful reading. The idea for this unique uniformed women's service sprang from the nimble brain of a Captain Baker on a battlefield in the Sudan campaign of 1898. Later, recounting the genesis of the FANY, he said:

> 'During my period of service with Lord Kitchener in the Sudan campaign, where I had the misfortune to be wounded, it occurred to me that there was a missing link somewhere in the Ambulance Department, which, in spite of the changes in warfare, had not altered very materially since the days of the Crimea when Florence Nightingale and her courageous band of helpers went out to succour and save the wounded. On my return from active service I thought out a plan which I anticipated would meet the want, but it was not until September, 1907, that I was able to found a troop of young women to see how my ideas on the subject would work.' (Irene Ward, *FANY Invicta*, London, 1955).

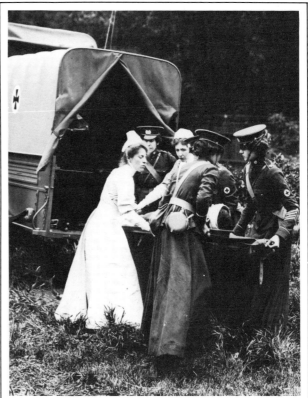

Members of the First Aid Nursing Yeomanry in training before the First World War practise loading a stretcher into a horse-drawn ambulance.

Captain Baker was a man of imagination and initiative. He conceived the idea of nurses galloping from field hospitals to the wounded on the battlefield, giving them first aid and remaining with them until the horse-drawn ambulance arrived. This explains why the corps started as a band of mounted nurses and also reveals the significance of the title First Aid Nursing Yeomanry.

By Sept. 1907, by means of an advertising campaign in the press, Captain Baker had assembled a body of young women with whom he could try out his ideas. In 1908 the constitution of the corps was drawn up, being registered in the following year. The FANY thus became the first women's voluntary corps to be organized in Britain, beating the Red Cross by a whisker, and they have maintained their voluntary status throughout their existence.

In the early days their recruits were mainly drawn from the upper-middle classes, although professional women subsequently made their own valuable contribution. In the beginning recruits owning their own horses were made particularly welcome. The FANY uniform was eye-catching. It consisted of a scarlet tunic with a high collar and white braid facings, a navy blue bell-shaped skirt with three rows of braid at the bottom, and a hard-topped scarlet cap with a shiny black peak, the whole outfit being completed with the addition of black patent leather riding boots, white gloves, a riding-crop and a first-aid kit in a haversack.

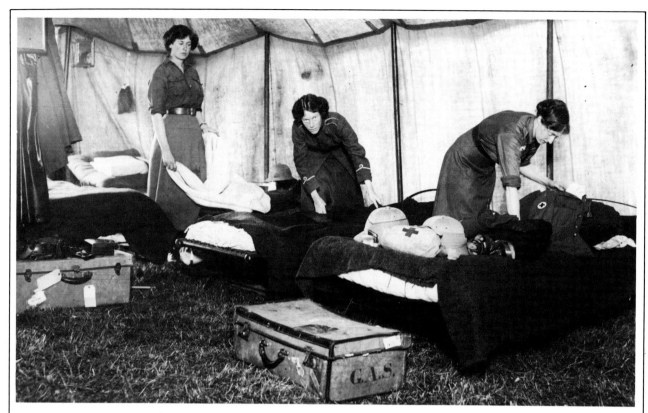

Women of the First Aid Nursing Yeomanry in camp at Pirbright, Surrey, in 1913 pack up their belongings before moving to fresh quarters.

On 1 Jan. 1916, after much stiff opposition from the War Office, official obstinacy was overcome, and the so-called 'Calais Convoy' came into being. For the first time in history women were officially employed as drivers for the British army. By the beginning of 1920 all the active service units of the corps had been demobilized, though many FANY were still working in France and Belgium, and even with the British Army of the Rhine.

However, after the First World War the FANY ceased to be nurses, the corps being subsequently trained as a mechanical transport unit. In 1938 the Army Council invited its cooperation in the formation of the Auxiliary Territorial Service. The unit now became the Women's Transport Service, supplying all personnel for the first ten driver companies of the ATS.

Royal nurses

On the outbreak of war great ladies rallied instantly to the call for arms, and the 80-year-old Empress Eugenie, widow of Napoleon III, gave a wing of her house, Farnborough Hill, as a convalescent home. There were three hospitals at Highgate superintended by the Grand Duchess George of Russia, assisted by her two daughters, the Princesses Xenia and Nina.

The wife of the Duke of Bedford, known as the 'Flying Duchess', was ready for all emergencies, as she had been trained in a London hospital in order to run the model hospital she founded at Woburn. It became a military hospital, and the doctors were glad of the help of the duchess, who had had further training in the duties of a surgeon's assistant radiologist.

Many of the ladies, such as the famous 'Flying Angels', who formed unofficial ambulance groups, were something of an embarrassment to the government, since they obeyed no rules but their own. One of these was the Dowager Duchess of Sutherland. Her aim was to get herself attached to the Secours aux Blessés, a branch of the French Red Cross, whose president happened to be a close friend of hers. While it was a strict rule that no foreigner should nurse in a French hospital, the duchess, flanked by the British ambassador in Paris, convinced the French minister of war that she was doing France a favour by bringing her distinguished person to its aid. Having broken every regulation to accede to her wishes, the minister gave the duchess a permit and offered his best wishes and warmest thanks as she set out with a party for Belgium.

There she immediately resigned from the Red Cross and, joining the Belgium Service de Santé, sent for and obtained the services of a surgeon and of eight trained nurses from England. However, no sooner had she and her doctor and nurses installed themselves than Namur was overrun by the

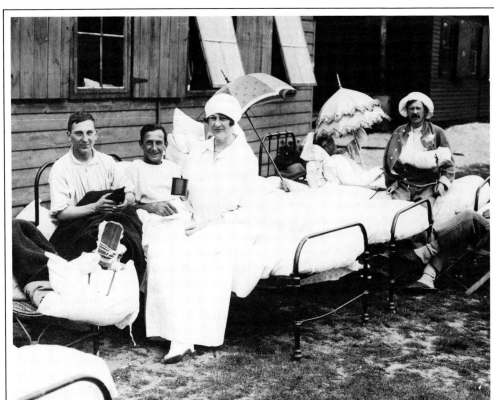

Left *The Duchess of Sutherland with wounded soldiers at her hospital at Calais in July 1917. The war brought people of different classes into close proximity with one another.*
Below *A ward in the Duchess of Westminster's hospital at Le Touquet in June 1917. During the war all kinds of buildings were requisitioned to serve as hospitals and beds were often crammed close together.*

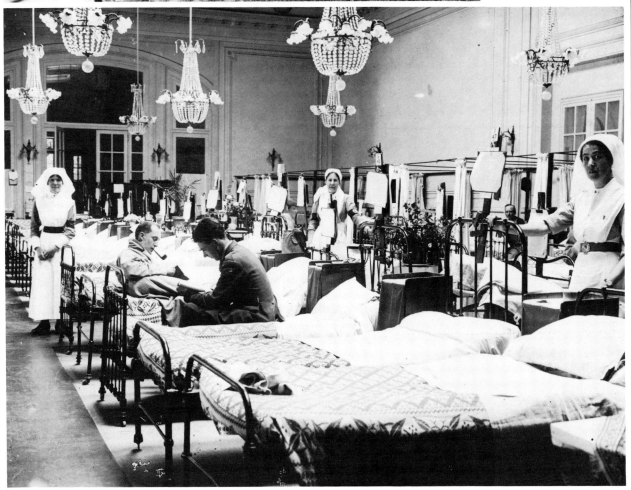

Opposite, above
Blinded soldiers and others with eye wounds at St Dunstan's Hospital, Regents Park, London, in 1914.
Opposite, below *A nurse attending a patient at a British military hospital in Rouen during the First World War.*
Right *Gassed soldiers, tended by a nurse, await their turn to be evacuated by ambulance. Many who survived gas attacks nevertheless remained lifelong invalids.*
Below *Nurses in France in June 1917 on board a hospital barge, a slow but effective way of transporting wounded men.*

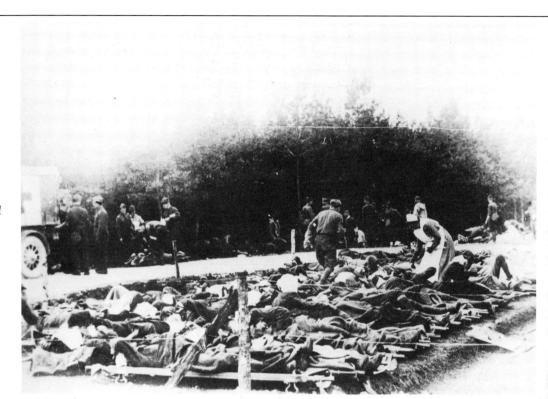

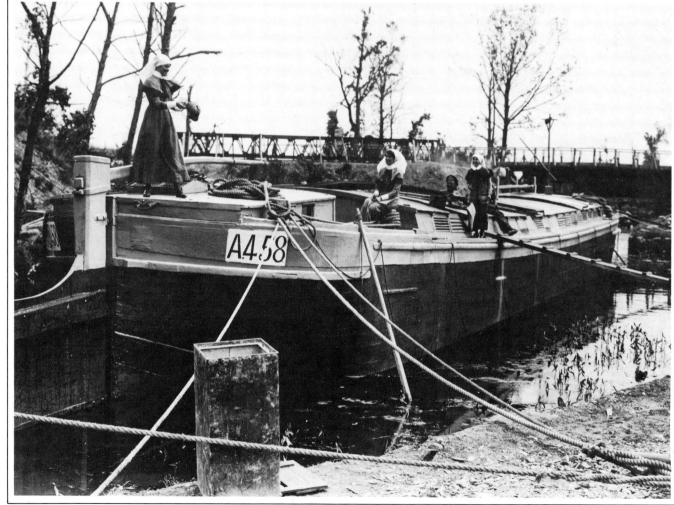

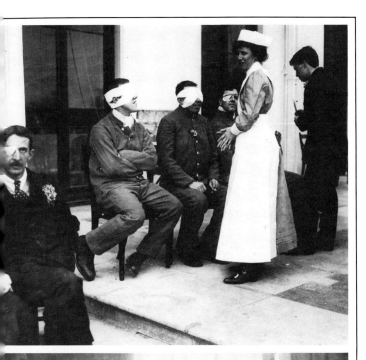

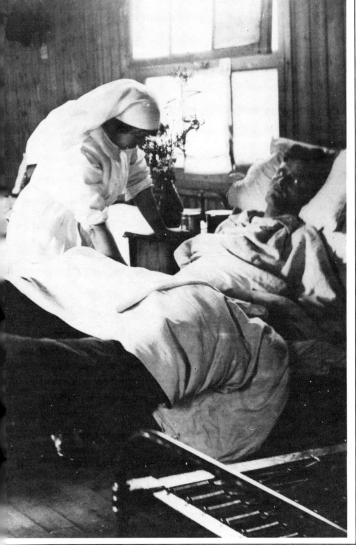

Germans. The people of Namur fled, but the Duchess remained at her post. She insisted on being addressed as 'Sister Millicent', and called daily upon the German authorities, pressing them for fresh supplies. Anxious to please a great English lady they obliged, while trying desperately to get her out of Belgium and into Holland. 'A more taxing operation,' said a German general, 'than many a military operation.'

In nearly every theatre of war some great lady would throw herself heart and soul into nursing. So it was with the Empress Alexandra of Russia. The vast Catherine Palace at Tsarskoe Selo was converted into a military hospital, and before the end of 1914 85 hospitals were operating under her patronage in Petrograd. Dressed in the simple grey uniform of a nursing sister, the empress, accompanied by two of her daughters, Olga and Tatiana, visited the hospital each day. 'I have seen the Empress of Russia in the operating theatre,' wrote one eye-witness, 'holding ether cones, handling sterilized instruments, assisting in the most difficult operations, taking from the hands of busy surgeons amputated arms and legs, removing the blood, even vermin-ridden field-dressings; enduring all the sights and smells and agonies of the most dreadful of all places, a military hospital in the midst of a war.'

Many remarkable women earned a distinguished place in the history of nursing during the First World War. Two of these, Lady Muriel Paget, with her deputy, Lady Sybil Grey, established a base hospital in Petrograd and field hospitals at several places on the eastern front during the years 1916 and 1917 when terrible casualties were being sustained by the Russian army. Lady Muriel Paget, the daughter of the 12th Earl of Winchelsea, had great personal courage and suffered all her life from chronic ill health. At the age of 39 she was inspired to form a unit of English surgeons and nurses as a gesture of good will towards the Russians, who offered her the Dimitri Palace in Petrograd, although it had its drawbacks as a hospital, since it had virtually no plumbing and the attics were occupied by old family retainers. The Grand Duke kept his own apartments, to which he returned from time to time from the front. The hospital, when completed, had accommodation for 180 beds, and the opening ceremony, a very grand affair, took place in Jan. 1916.

The Women's Hospital Corps

At the outbreak of war two outstanding women doctors, Louisa Garrett Anderson (daughter of the great Elizabeth Garrett Anderson) and Flora Murray were determined that women physicians wishing to give their services to the nation should not be excluded from work with the armed forces.

Knowing they would receive short shrift from the War Office, the two enterprising ladies went quietly to the French Embassy and laid their case before a somewhat puzzled

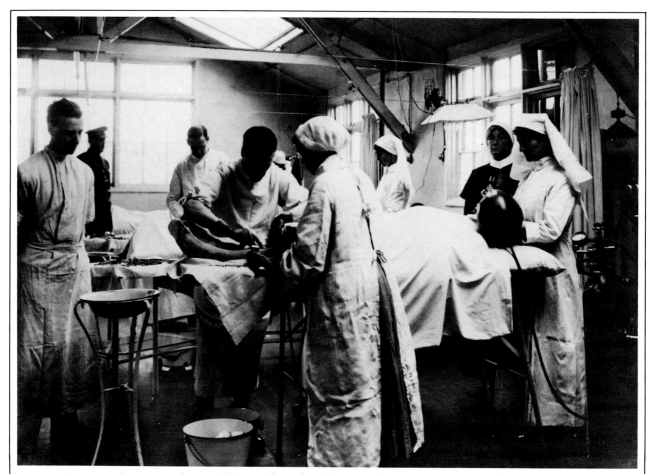

A scene in the operating theatre at Wimereux hospital, which was run by two British women doctors, Louisa Garrett Anderson and Flora Murray.

official who sent them on to Madame Brasier du Thuy, president of the branch of the French Red Cross known as L'Union des Femmes de France. She was working hard to raise money and comforts for the French Red Cross, and welcomed the two doctors with open arms. She was delighted with their offer of a fully equipped surgical unit composed of women doctors and trained nurses. The offer of the British doctors was transmitted to higher authority, and within a week a formal acceptance from Paris reached Dr Garrett Anderson, accompanied by a request that the unit be organized immediately and be ready if required to begin work on 1 Dec. 1914.

On 14 Sept. 1914 the Women's Hospital Corps left Victoria for Paris. It had been decided that they should open a hospital in the Hotel Claridge, which had been placed at the disposal of the French Red Cross. The hotel, a large modern building on the Champs-Elysées, had just been completed and was still full of workmen cleaning up the debris. The doctors concluded that they would be able to receive 100 patients. Everyone turned to and began cleaning the place and preparing it for the wounded.

The first visitor was a doctor from the American Hospital. At the outbreak of the war the American colony in Paris had organized a superb hospital in the Lycée at Neuilly and had established a fleet of ambulances. These carried hundreds of wounded men from the front to Paris. Both French and British wounded were in desperate straits since at that time there was no organized motor transport service, and the armies depended on the railways for the removal of the sick and injured.

The American doctor, who had more patients than he could cope with, had come to see whether the British doctors might be willing to take some of his cases in their hospital. Dr Murray rose to the occasion. Oblivious of the chaos around her, she said with conviction, 'We can take 24 this afternoon, and another 26 tonight.'

So successful was the hospital that the two British doctors were asked to open another one at Wimereux. This, too, was considered to be a great success, but in the course of time the cases coming down to the base were medical cases or had slight injuries which made their early transfer to England possible. Thus the work at the hospital at Wimereux assumed more and more the character of a clearing station.

It was at this point that Doctors Garrett Anderson and Murray were summoned to England for an interview with the director-general of Army Medical Services, Sir Alfred

Keogh. He asked them to close their unit in France and bring it to London, offering them charge of a hospital of 500 or a 1000 beds. The staff was to consist of women, and the task of finding additional doctors and nurses was to rest with the organizers.

The old workhouse in St Giles, Bloomsbury, had been taken over by the War Office for hospital purposes, and it was there that Sir Alfred Keogh decided to station the Women's Hospital Corps. The group of buildings was at the upper end of Endell Street, on ground granted by Queen Matilda as a lepers' hospital. Part of the administrative block bore the date 1727, and St Giles was said to have been the workhouse described by Dickens in *Oliver Twist*.

The first matron was a Miss Hale, at that time matron of the Elizabeth Garrett Anderson Hospital and a member of the Territorial Force Nursing Service. Some of the sisters from the French hospital continued as members of the Corps.

The hospital, designed to accommodate 520 cases, consisted of 17 wards, of which three smaller ones were reserved for severe cases. Of the 26,000 patients who passed through its wards, the greatest number were British, with a good proportion of Dominion and colonial troops.

In Oct. 1919 an order was issued to evacuate and close the hospital, but the doctors had made their case. Through their initiative and efficiency they provided many more future opportunities for women physicians, surgeons and members of the nursing profession.

Edith Cavell

It would be impossible to write about nursing in World War I without mentioning the name of Edith Cavell. Born in 1865, when she was 30 she went to the London Hospital as a probationer and subsequently nursed in England for some years, before moving to Brussels. In 1907 she was appointed matron of the Berkendael Medical Institute in Brussels, which she transformed from a small clinic into a teaching hospital with an international reputation.

When in 1914 the German army invaded Belgium, she remained at her post to care for the sick and wounded sent to her clinic, which had become a Red Cross hospital. She continued to give sanctuary to wounded fighting men of all nationalities and for eight months the hospital became a staging post on the escape route for hundreds of Allied soldiers. At the same time, with the calm that characterized her, she continued with her nursing duties.

In Aug. 1915 she was arrested for harbouring enemy aliens and helping them to escape. Sentenced to death, she was, despite the efforts of neutral diplomats, executed by a firing squad in Oct. 1915. Nurse Cavell met her death with unflinching courage. Her last message was:

'Standing as I do in view of God and Eternity, I realise that patriotism is not enough. I must have no hatred or bitterness towards anyone.'

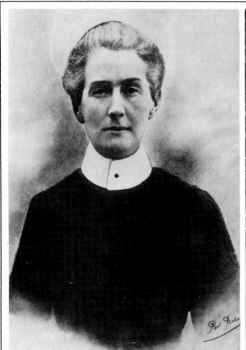

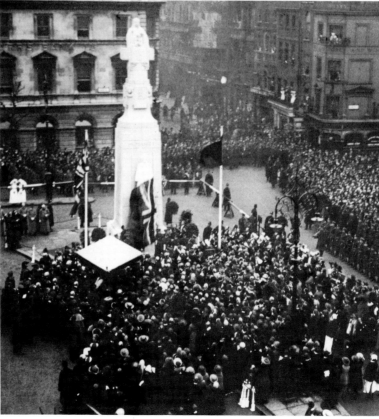

Above *Edith Cavell. Her execution by the German occupation authorities in Brussels provoked a storm of indignation in Britain.* **Right** *The unveiling of her statue in London in March 1920.*

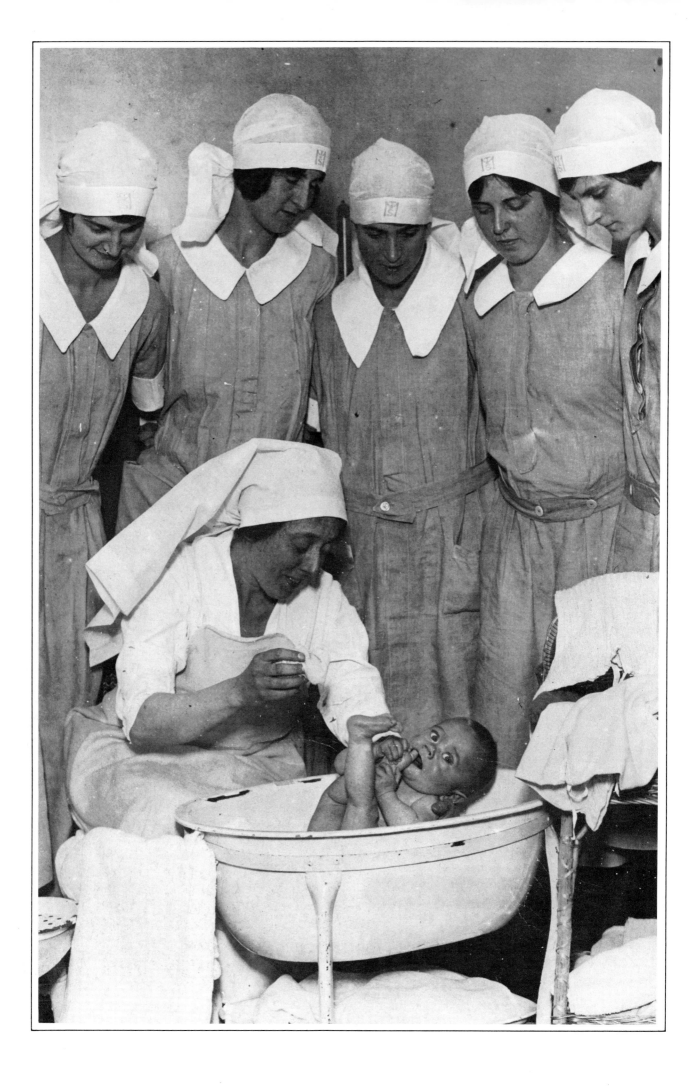

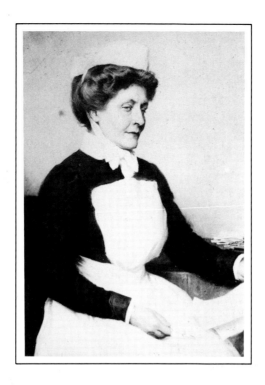

The Royal College of Nursing

Towards a College of Nursing

The war had taken a terrible toll. Some ten million men of all nations had been killed, most of them under the age of 40, while twice that number had been wounded and a considerable proportion maimed for life. Women had taken over work previously done only by men. They took their place on the land, in shops, offices, factories, voluntary services, schools and hospitals. Modern warfare had demanded a total national effort and the women of Great Britain played their part. The militant group who had agitated for emancipation were jubilant, but made it clear that once the war was over, women should not fade into the background. Indeed, by the time peace was declared, the emancipation of women was practically a fait accompli, and in 1918, with hardly a dissenting voice, women over 30 in Britain were given the vote. This was a great step forward, but it soon became evident that the aftermath of war was going to pose a great many problems which would affect not only the men returning from the front, but also the male orderlies, the VADs and the nursing profession in general.

Much had been said and written about the recruitment, training and education of nurses. It was, however, 'a profession without any really representative organization, effec-

tive in nature, even including Ethel Bedford Fenwick's RBNA'. How then were nurses going to cope with the peacetime world? How would the 'emancipated' woman consolidate her new status? To whom would she look for guidance? Before the First World War nursing had no dominant organization to whom all members of the profession could turn for leadership, representation and help.

It was Sarah Swift who was to find a solution to the problems which had so long beset nursing. Retiring after 20 years as matron of Guy's Hospital in 1909, she determined to rescue nursing from the chaotic state in which it found itself. Having formulated a plan of campaign, she sought an interview with Arthur Stanley, chairman of the British section of the Red Cross. She proposed the formation of an effective central body – a College of Nursing – modelled to some extent on the College of Physicians and Surgeons. By the time the interview was over, Stanley had promised Sarah Swift his full support.

Both knew that a tough battle lay ahead of them, for the guidelines she wanted to lay down were bound to meet with great opposition, not only from Mrs Ethel Bedford Fenwick, self-styled leader of the nursing profession, but possibly also from the legendary Florence Nightingale who was still alive.

What Sarah Swift proposed was a rational and practical approach to the problem. She wanted registration of bona fide nurses of good character irrespective of social origins. She wanted a standardized system of training laid down with a written examination to follow, in which educational attainments were to be subordinate to technical knowledge.

Both Sarah Swift and Arthur Stanley had a highly developed sense of occasion, and they decided to organize a

Top Dame Sarah Swift, matron of Guy's Hospital 1901–09 and founder of the Royal College of Nursing.
Opposite Nurses at a mothercraft class in the 1920s being shown how to bath a baby.

luncheon party to which they would invite the people they thought might give strong support to their great project.

History does not relate the exact circumstances of this meal, but there is no doubt that the guests were admirably chosen and would, each in their own way, make an important contribution to the founding in the College of Nursing.

Apart from Arthur Stanley, the only other man actively involved in the project at the time was Cooper Perry, Medical Superintendent of Guy's Hospital, a man with a dazzling academic background, and whose powers of organization and administration were used for the betterment of suffering humanity. The other two women at the luncheon party were also remarkable in their own way and in their own field.

Rachael Annie Cox-Davies, like Sarah Swift, had a strong personality and an impressive nursing background. Alicia Lloyd Still was one of Florence Nightingale's personally chosen trainees at the Nightingale Training School. Like her two colleagues, she was a woman of outstanding ability, and rose to the top of her profession. It was she who invented the office of 'Sister Tutor' in 1913 when, having reorganized the Training School at St Thomas' and produced a new curriculum for a three-year course, she placed a sister in charge of all instruction.

All three women were to end their careers heaped with honours, and all three during their working lives were formidable disciplinarians who expected and exacted the highest standards of the nurses under them.

The founding of the Royal College of Nursing

It was not long before a number of outstanding personalities in the medical world became interested in the idea of a College of Nursing. One of these was the gynaecologist, Comyns Berkeley. From the outset he was an enthusiastic and helpful supporter of Sarah Swift's efforts. A member of the first council, he was appointed the first honorary treasurer, an appointment he held until his death in 1946.

On 27 March 1916, the College of Nursing was registered as a limited company. Its main objectives were:

1. To promote the better education and training of nurses and the advancement of nursing as a profession in all or any of its branches.

2. To promote uniformity of curriculum.

3. To recognize approved nursing schools.

4. To make and maintain a register of persons to whom certificates of proficiency or of training and proficiency had been granted.

5. To promote Bills in Parliament for any object connected with the interests of the nursing profession and, in particular, with nurse education, organization, protection, or for their recognition by the state.

Initially, nurses applying for entry to the college register were required to have had training in civil hospitals or infirmaries with at least 250 beds and with a resident medical or surgical officer. At least one course of lectures per annum must have been given and a final examination held before certificates were issued.

Until the College acquired its own premises, the council meetings were held at the Royal Automobile Club in Pall Mall, which became the official registered office.

A sub-committee was appointed to meet representatives of various societies for state registration, and training schools were invited to send representatives to a meeting to discuss the formation of a consultative board. At the fourth council meeting Mary Rundle was appointed secretary, an inspired choice which was to lead to 17 years of selfless dedication in forwarding the affairs of the College and nursing in general.

The sudden and tragic death of Mary Rundle's fiancé had decided her to devote her life to nursing and, after training at St Bartholomew's Hospital, she went to New York where she took a course in hospital economics, and also studied teaching methods and curricula in various American nurse-training schools.

On returning to England she held many important posts. In 1912 she was appointed matron of the Royal Hospital for Diseases of the Chest, and in 1915 she became matron of the London General Hospital, Territorial Army Nursing Service, and was later awarded the Royal Cross.

Mary Rundle had flair and initiative and organized some of the earliest post-graduate courses for nurses on tuberculosis nursing and health visiting and began her own nursing library. Her most important work was in helping to initiate a superannuation scheme for nurses and hospital officers.

Sharing Mary Rundle's dedication to her work was her colleague and friend, Gertrude Cowlin, who joined her as assistant secretary of the College of Nursing in 1917. She was to be in turn registrar, organizing secretary of the local centres, chief of the information bureau and librarian. In 1924 she added the job of education officer as well as that of librarian. She was subsequently appointed editor of the *Nursing Times*.

Gertrude Cowlin was also the first librarian of the Library of Nursing which was established from a grant from the Carnegie United Kingdom Trust, and it was she who collected the nucleus of what is believed to be the finest nursing library in the world.

At the first ordinary general meeting of the College of Nursing on 18 May 1916, the chairman was able to announce that over 70 training schools and societies had replied to the letters he had sent them and had nominated representatives to the consultative board. This was followed by a meeting with representatives of the various societies for the state registration of nurses to confer with the legal registration committee of the College.

With the adoption of the report, the first official year in the life of the College came to a close. So successful was the idea of the College that at the next ordinary general meet-

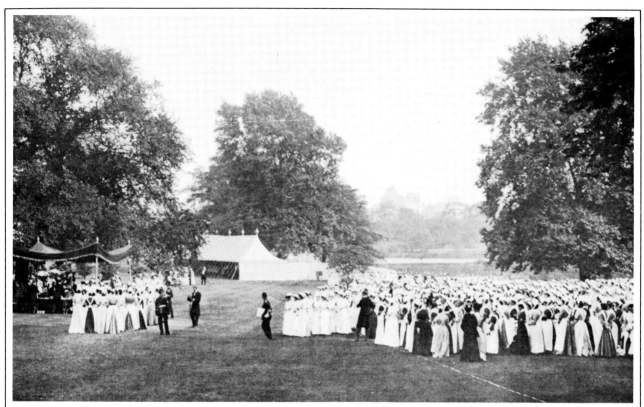

Queen Alexandra receiving members of the Nurses' Royal Pension Fund at Buckingham Palace in July 1904. The queen always took a keen interest in all aspects of nursing.

ing, a year later, the chairman was able to announce a nurse membership of over 7000.

Although the College attracted nurse-membership from all over the British Empire, it was not nearly so successful in getting an agreement on terms for state registration. The central committee for the state registration of trained nurses had prepared and presented a bill to Parliament and would not agree to the amendments to certain clauses made by the College committee. Obstinate as ever, Mrs Bedford Fenwick refused to give in or even to compromise. Finally the central committee's bill was rejected by Parliament.

Although Mrs Bedford Fenwick had done a great deal to further the advancement of the nursing profession, she considered the College and everyone connected with it as inimical to herself. Since it had not been her brainchild, she would have no truck with it, and attacked its aims whenever possible.

Donations began to come in at a satisfactory rate for the College, which raised the spirits of those working in cramped conditions in the tiny office in Vere Street, London. Both the College council and the Royal British Nurses Association were quick to see that it would be advantageous to both parties if they amalgamated. As soon as Mrs Bedford Fenwick learnt about this possibility, although no longer persona grata with the RBNA, she tried diligently to squash the idea. Eventually the RBNA lost interest in amalgamating with the College and the matter was finally dropped.

State registration

In the meantime discussions had gone on with the central committee for the state registration of nurses, but Mrs Bedford Fenwick was still refusing to accept any changes. Eventually, however, after prolonged discussions, the matter was taken out of the hands of the nursing profession by the administrator of the newly created Ministry of Health (previously a local government department). The bill was redrafted and, as a result, the Nurses Act finally received the Royal Assent, and passed into law on 23 Dec. 1919. It contained the provisions for training and registration already agreed upon by the two main bodies but, most important of all, it also contained the requirements insisted upon by the College against all opposition that a minimum of two-thirds of the General Nursing Council be democratically elected by nurses on the National Register.

In the early part of 1920 the minister of health invited the College to submit names for its representatives on the first General Nursing Council established under the terms of the Act. The College obtained these by postal vote from the nurses on its own register. Those elected were Miss Cox-Davies, Miss Lloyd Still, and Miss Sparshott. The new General Nursing Council for England and Wales had the duty to form and keep a register of nurses for the sick consisting of the following parts:

A general part containing the names of all nurses qualifying according to details to be laid down by the General Nursing Council.

A supplementary part containing the names of male nurses.

A supplementary part containing the names of mental nurses.

A supplementary part containing the names of nurses trained in the nursing of sick children.

All rules concerning training qualification and admission to the register had to be approved by the minister of health, and there were also details for the registration of 'existing nurses' who had been in practice for a minimum of three years prior to Nov. 1919, and whom the GNC regarded as 'having adequate knowledge and experience of nursing the sick'. There were penalties for any who unlawfully assumed the title of 'registered nurse' or who gave false information in applying for registration.

Similar acts were shortly passed to cover Scotland and Ireland. These acts together formed the most important measures for the protection of the public from the untrained and ignorant and also, for the first time, put the nursing profession upon a proper basis as regards training and qualifi-

cation. Mrs Bedford Fenwick, however, refused to acknowledge defeat, and through the columns of her *British Journal of Nursing* strongly opposed the concept of state registration. She attacked the register, which she said would be 'flooded by VADs, village nurses and cottage nurses who have shirked training'.

Whatever her feelings on the subject, nurses were in demand and the passage of time would deal with all her objections. In the meantime Parliament overrode the General Nursing Council and made it possible for nurses to be admitted to the register providing they could present three certificates attesting to their good character and competence.

In Jan. 1919, the College of Nursing had moved to No. 7 Henrietta Street (later renamed Henrietta Place), Cavendish Square. It was soon evident, however, that a new headquarters would be needed to house an administrative organization that was growing daily. Rachael Cox-Davies was determined that, somehow or other, she would raise sufficient funds to finance a purpose-built college which would have room to incorporate all the facilities that were needed for present and future developments.

It was her connection with the generous and wealthy Lady Cowdray which made her dream possible. Lady Cowdray had always displayed an active interest in all aspects of nursing,

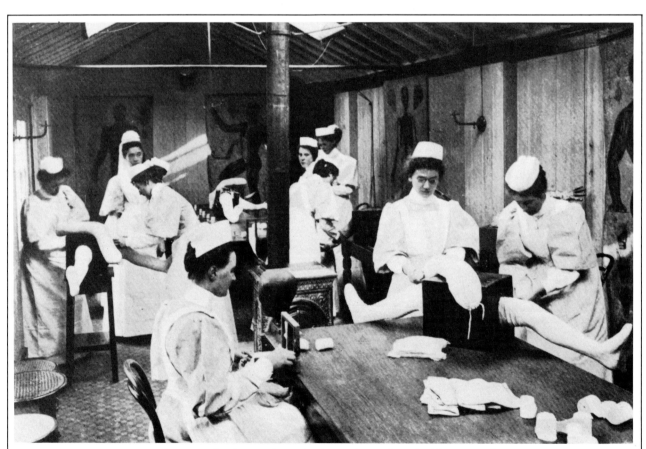

Nurses under training busily at work in a bandaging class at the end of the nineteenth century.

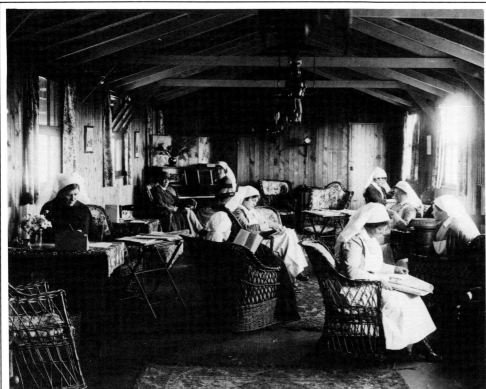

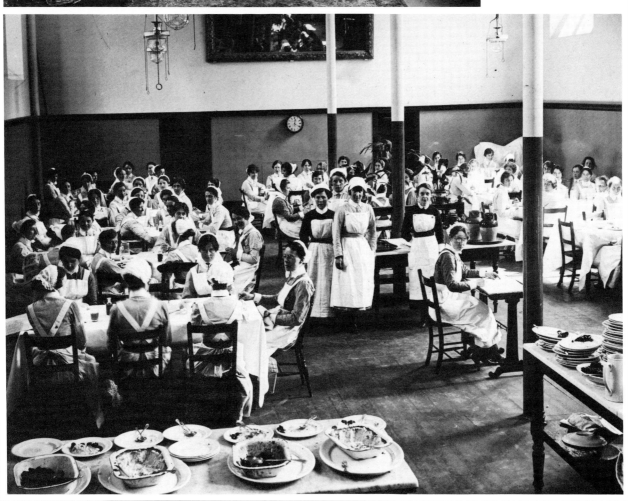

Left *Nurses relaxing at the Princess Victoria Rest Club for Nurses at Etaples, France, in 1917.*
Below *At lunch in the dining hall at St Bartholomew's Hospital in 1921.*

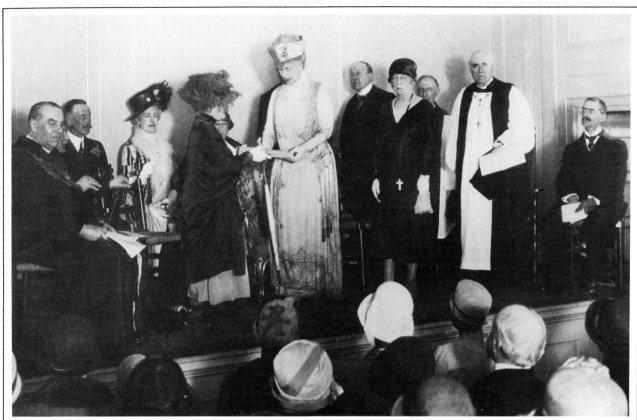

The opening of Cowdray Hall, the new headquarters of the Royal College of Nursing, in May 1926. Queen Mary is presenting the deeds to Dame Sarah Swift. Seated at the far right is Neville Chamberlain, then minister of health.

had already provided two sister-tutor studentships for College members, and in 1921 was elected to the council of the College.

Lady Cowdray did not fail Rachael Cox-Davies. She made £500,000 available to the College, and this sum was used to purchase the splendid mansion on the corner of Henrietta Place and Cavendish Square, which had been the London home of the former prime minister, Herbert Asquith.

Extensive renovations took place, and the house was converted into a residential club for nurses and professional women called the Cowdray Club. The garden of the club fronted Henrietta Place, and it was here that it was hoped to build the new college headquarters. The Cowdray Club was opened on 2 June 1922 by Lady Cowdray, who on the same occasion laid the foundation stone for what was to be the new headquarters of the College of Nursing. This was eventually opened on 21 May 1926 by Queen Mary. It was a grand occasion with a spectacular guard of honour lining the entrance, whose members had been drawn from the nursing services of the Crown, the hospitals and public health and domiciliary nurses from all parts of the country.

However, there was one person who did not share in the general rejoicing. This was Ethel Bedford Fenwick, who had, that very same year, launched the rival British College of Nursing, an endowment believed to be sponsored by one of her husband's grateful patients. Although it carried on for many years, it was always overshadowed by the College of Nursing, which had the distinction of having Queen Mary as its first patron. She always took a keen interest in the College and was a frequent visitor.

Nursing conditions

Within two years of its foundation the College undertook a survey of the conditions of work and salaries of nurses. Its findings were horrifying. The College then published what was to become known as the 'Nurses' Charter'. It was sent out to all nurse-employing authorities, with the request that improvements in salary scales and working conditions should be adopted without delay. Some local authorities and hospitals complied, but there were many who refused to make any concessions and the College pursued them vigorously down the years until the founding of the National Health Service.

In June 1926 a proposal to apply for a Royal Charter was mooted, and the following year a draft charter and petition were submitted. The petition set out the aims and objects of the College, its financial position and its achievements. It now had a membership of over 26,000, and the support of a number of training schools and other auxiliary professional organizations. In June 1928 'His Majesty in Council was pleased to approve the grant of a charter to the College of Nursing.' However, it was not until 11 years later that the title 'royal' was incorporated in the charter, this honour being granted by King George VI.

The one issue on which the various professional organizations agreed was that there must be only one method of entry to the nursing profession. With the exception of fever nurses, only those who had undergone a three-year training in a hospital should be allowed to bear the title nurse. As early as 1905, however, the select committee on registration had suggested there might be a need for a separate register for nurses whose training was of a lower standard than that laid down for registered nurses but, because of the fear that the VADs, so unpopular with registered nurses, might take this short cut to becoming recognized nurses, the idea of a separate register was eventually rejected. Though the vexed question of 'assistant nurses' was to crop up again and again, it was not until the Nurses Act of 1949 that statutory recognition was given to assistant nurses.

One of the major problems that had always bedevilled the nursing profession was that there were two schools of thought about the education of nurses. From the time of Florence Nightingale it was taken for granted both by her and by her disciples that there were two kinds of nurse: the young girl of good family destined for executive office, and the more humble creature, a country girl, housekeeper or widow, who did not need higher education to carry out the simple tasks demanded of a well-disciplined nurse.

The second school of thought believed otherwise. It was their contention that all nurses, no matter what their background, should be educated up to a certain standard, after which, if they wanted higher education, they should be entitled to have it.

It was, therefore, the task of the College to set up an Education Department with links with universities. It was agreed that the most vital need was to educate the teachers of nurses and, already in 1918, courses were arranged with Bedford College and with the University of London which awarded a diploma in nursing.

Nurses were now branching out in all directions, and those working in specialized fields needed specialist teaching. There were nurses in factories, schools, in all branches of public health and overseas, where both the English nurse and English teaching methods were in great demand.

As far back as 1878, the first industrial nurse was appointed by the firm of J. and J. Colman, of mustard fame, in Norwich. Nurse Philippa Flowerday, then aged 32, had trained for a year at the Norfolk and Norwich Hospital before going to Colman's Carrow Works. She was engaged by Caroline Colman, wife of the senior partner, at 26 shillings a week, 'on condition of her father's moving to live near Carrow as soon as we can find a suitable cottage'.

Nurse Flowerday started each day at Carrow in the dispensary where she helped the doctor. At mid-morning she loaded up a basket of supplies from the Carrow Works

kitchen and set off to see the sick in their homes, making about 45 visits a week. She co-operated with Colman's Sick Benefit Society which administered a clothing club and lending library, and helped distribute Christmas presents. She was not expected to do night duty and had her Sundays free. In 1888 Nurse Flowerday left the Carrow Works to marry William Reid, Colman's head gardener at their seaside home near Lowestoft. That same year, Sister Quarry, who had trained at St Mary's Hospital, Paddington, took Nurse Flowerday's place. The pattern was then set for an industrial

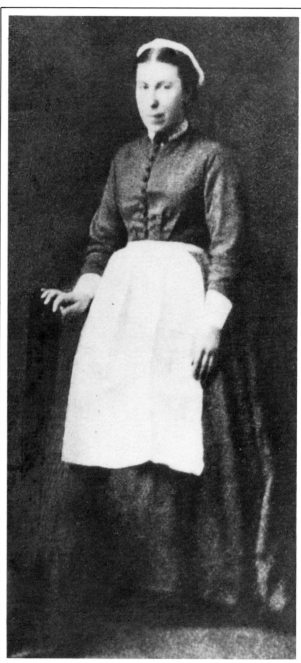

Philippa Flowerday, the first known industrial nurse, was appointed in 1878 by J. and J. Coleman to look after the health of their employees.

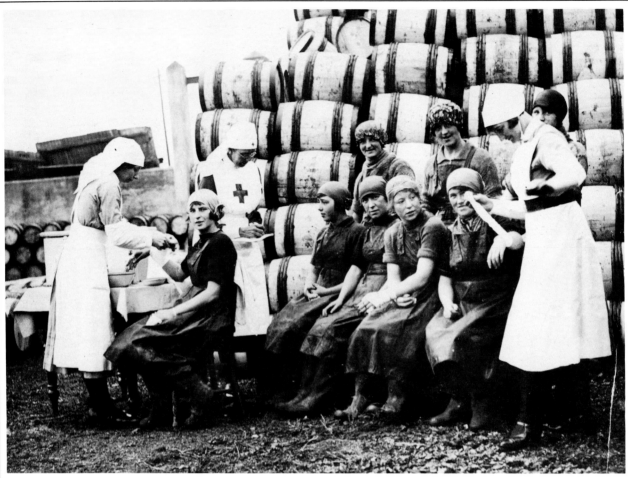

Red Cross nurses banding the hands of fisher girls at Great Yarmouth, Norfolk, in the 1920s. In the twentieth century increasing attention was being given to occupational health.

nurse always to be appointed to the firm of Colman, and their example was followed by a number of companies, who were quick to see the benefits of having a trained nurse-cum-health visitor on their payroll.

Male nurses

Already in 1901 the profession was being quietly infiltrated by male nurses. The census of population of this year reported that there were in fact about 6000 male nurses. By 1921 there were over 11,000, and by 1931 over 15,000. They were, however, employed almost exclusively in mental hospitals and as mental nurses in private homes. Their only firm niche in general hospitals was the care of male patients with venereal disease. The prejudices against male nurses were to be found in the attitude of the militantly feminist nurses, who thought they would not be able to order male nurses about as easily as the more docile females. There was also the fear that male nurses might make sexual advances towards their female colleagues. Even more deep rooted

among the matrons was the anxiety that male nurses might well be homosexual and thus create difficult situations with the patients.

As late as 1937 there were less than 100 male nurses at work in the voluntary hospitals, although the local authorities had fewer qualms and some of them opened up training facilities for men. Even so, in 1937 all the authorities in England and Wales only employed a total of approximately 1500 male nurses, most of whom were unqualified.

At a time of high unemployment in the 1930s a good many men went into psychiatric nursing. After the outbreak of war, a large number of men were to work as orderlies in the Royal Army Medical Corps, and in the postwar period some of them decided to continue their work and become more recognized in general nursing. The first overall register for male nurses, however, was not established until 1949, and it was only during the late 1950s and the 1960s that men achieved greater recognition in general nursing. Though at first they always nursed their own sex, in recent years male midwives have been allowed to practise. Interestingly enough, both male and female nurses have the same wage structure.

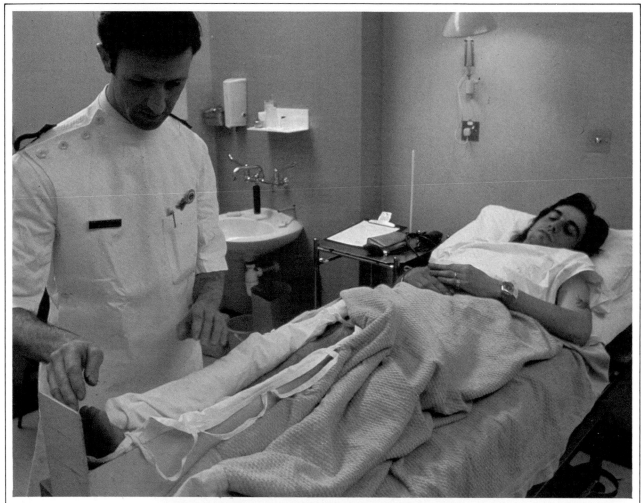

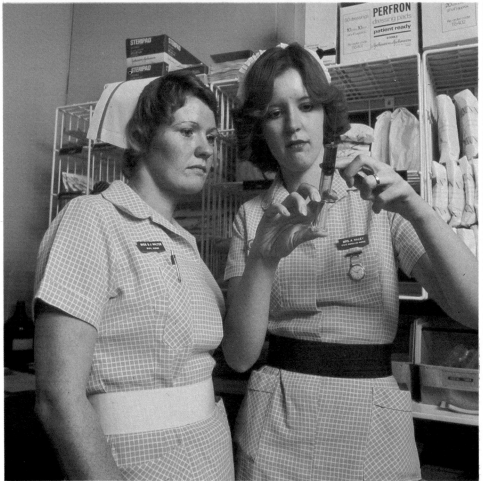

Above A male nurse attending to a patient with his leg in plaster. In recent years changes in the career structure of nursing have enabled men to attain high positions in the profession.
Right A staff nurse demonstrates the use of a hypodermic to a student nurse.

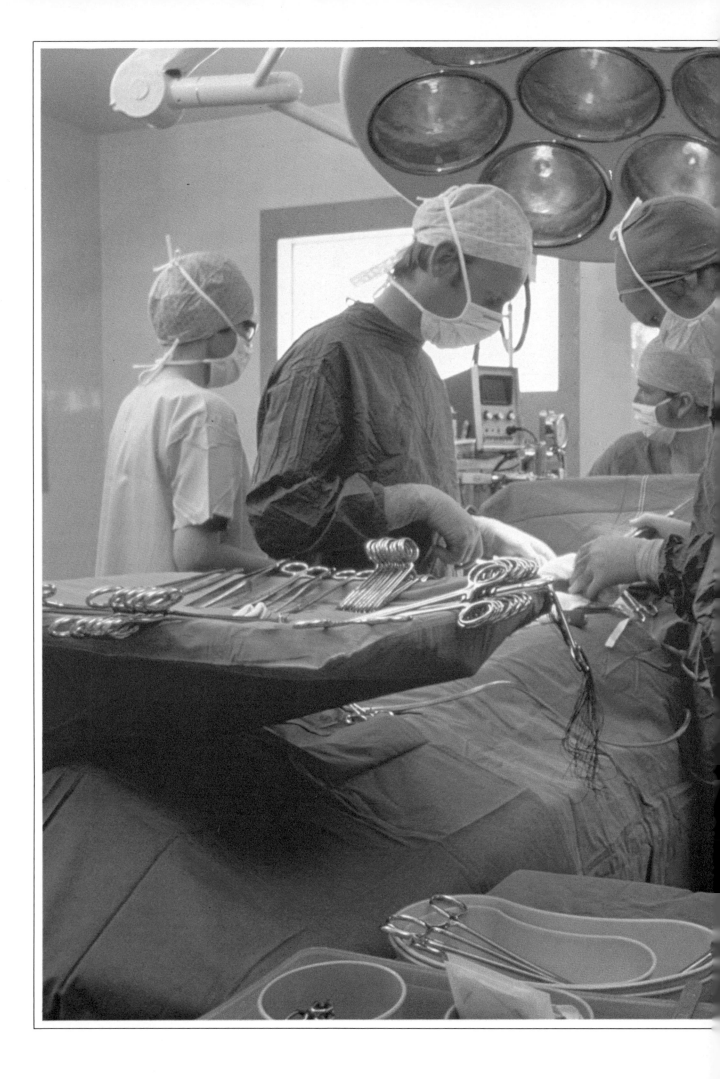

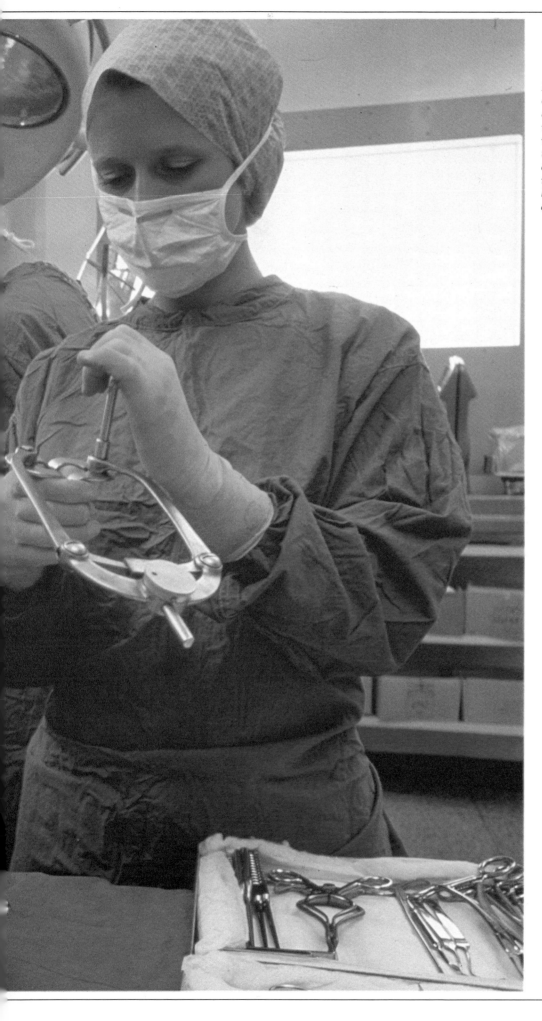

Nurses at work in an operating theatre. The enormous advances in medical knowledge in recent years have meant that nurses have constantly had to acquire new skills in order to keep abreast of developments.

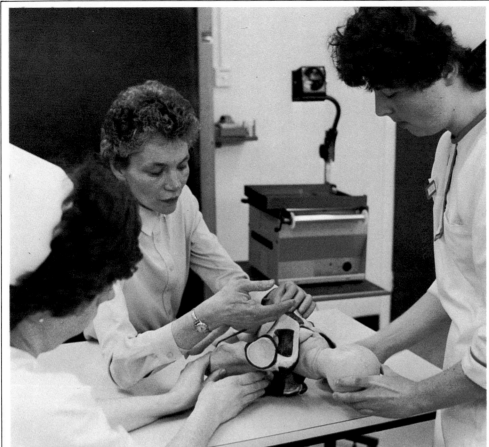

Left Student midwives undergoing instruction with the use of a dummy. Midwifery training combines theory and practice at every stage.
Below A young mother looks on while a community midwife weighs the baby. Community midwives are responsible for providing ante- and post-natal care as well as for conducting deliveries that take place at home.

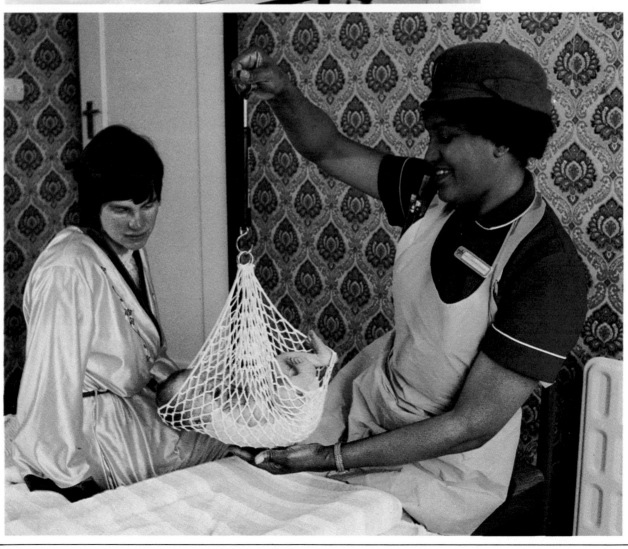

Another landmark was when the Royal College of Nursing accepted men into membership in 1961, an almost unbelievable break with tradition. Over the last 20 years, although the proportion of male nurses to female nurses has remained about 10%, men have carved out important careers for themselves in nursing, and have reached eminent senior positions, both in management and education.

Uniforms

There was no detail too small to be overlooked by those who had the reputation of the British state registered nurse to heart. It was decided – after much deliberation – in Feb. 1921 that the seal to be used on every registration certificate was to be a medallion, with Hygeia (the Goddess of Health) in the centre, the rose of England on the right, the daffodil of Wales on the left, together with a scroll with 'A.D. 1919' inscribed on it and, round the margin, the title 'The General Nursing Council for England and Wales'. The Scottish seal incorporated the cross of St Andrew, and the Irish medallion a leaf of shamrock in each corner.

There were also lengthy debates on the uniform to be worn by nurses. It was finally agreed as follows:

Skirt not to be less than eight inches and not more than twelve inches from the ground; or coat frock with small detachable cape for outdoor wear. The material to be of two weights, and navy-blue in colour: for summer wear, shower-proof gabardine, for winter wear serge. Buttons, bone with Tudor rose in the centre and the lettering 'England and Wales' round. Braid – artificial silk in navy with royal blue centre.

Hat – for winter wear, velour (blue). For summer straw (blue). Trimming – navy blue ribbon with woven badge similar to badge chosen. Storm cap – of same material as coat, with braiding on flat, and woven badge in front. Shoes: Black or tan. Stockings: black, tan or grey. Gloves: Tan, grey or white.

Shirt to be worn with coat and skirt. White silk or cotton with polo collar fitting up the neck. Tie: Blue Irish poplin (same colour as centre of braiding).

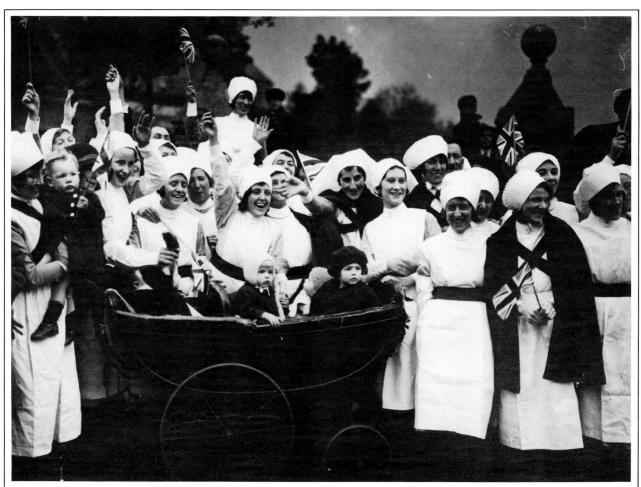

Nurses with their charges provide an enthusiastic welcome for Queen Mary as she arrives to open the Middlesex County Hospital extension at Isleworth in Feb. 1932.

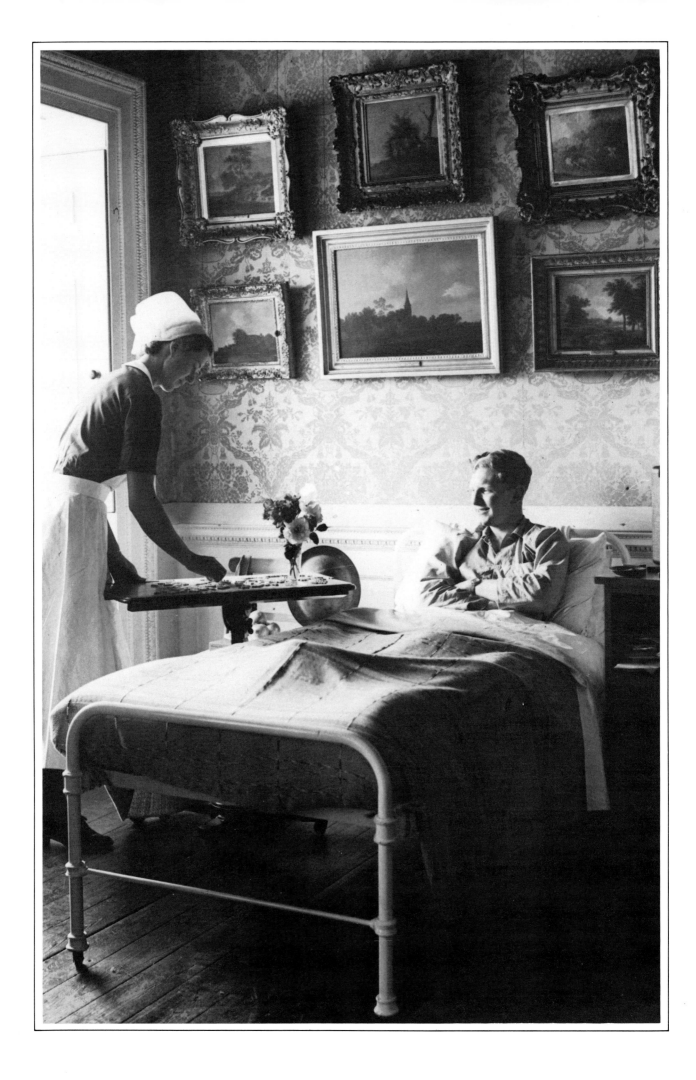

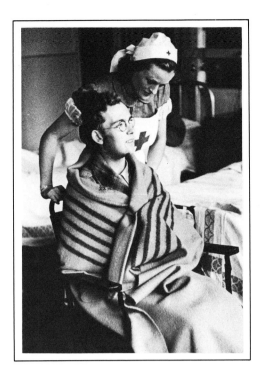

The fight for better conditions and the advent of the Second World War

The status of nurses

At the beginning of the twentieth century nurses had received much the same pay in local and voluntary hospital sectors. Both wages and conditions of work were unsatisfactory and, although an endless succession of committees submitted reports demanding radical changes, their recommendations were never properly implemented, 'nursing being one of the professions subject to the greatest number of reports whose recommendations have led to the least action.'

In 1930 the pay of probationers in voluntary hospitals averaged £20 in the first year, £25 in the second and £30 in the third. Municipal hospitals were slightly more generous, but in this same year staff nurses in training schools started off with the princely wage of £52.55, while voluntary and municipal hospitals paid ten pounds a year more.

In 1937 the pay in voluntary hospitals was almost the same as it had been in 1930, although the local authorities gave probationers more. The nurses were paid in cash and provided with free board and lodgings of a spartan simplicity.

In 1930 and 1937 nurses employed in local authority hospitals worked shorter hours than in voluntary hospitals, in which nursing staff averaged approximately 117 hours a fortnight in London, and 119 hours a fortnight in the provinces. In municipal hospitals, however, the hours were less – only 113 hours a fortnight.

Over the years, beginning with the haloed image of Florence Nightingale gliding around hushed and adoring wards with her lamp, the nursing profession had been glamorized and romanticized in novels, plays and later in films. Pain and suffering and the realities of illness were kept well in the background.

However, in nursing, fact is infinitely stranger than fiction, and infinitely bloodier too. The young women who took up nursing in the 1930s soon had their rose-coloured spectacles knocked off their noses by their starched and disciplined elders, who put them through a course of training which either confirmed their desire to stay in nursing or sent them scurrying off to look for a less taxing occupation.

Glimpses of what nursing is really about can be found in the pages of any number of diaries and autobiographies. One of these, *A Nurse in Time* by Evelyn Prentis, gave an accurate picture of what life as a probationer was like in an English hospital in 1934.

Top *A Red Cross nurse with a patient in a wheelchair in 1941. The various nursing services were better organized in the Second World War than they had been in 1914.*
Opposite *Still confined to bed, an army officer at Harewood House, the residence of the Princess Royal, which had been converted into a convalescent home for sick and wounded soldiers for the duration of the war.*

'As at school we learned many things we would never need to know and were left in ignorance of things that might well have been useful to us. . . . We earnestly studied the conversion of mare's milk into human milk, though for what purpose was never made clear. We learned how to put leeches on and how to drop salt on their tails to make them get off again. . . . We put things into patients and took things out of them. We poulticed, purged, plastered and posseted.'

Evelyn Prentis had a loving heart and great powers of observation. In her book she talked sadly of rickety and under-nourished and dying children in the wards.

'We splinted their limbs, straightened their spines, forced milk into them, choked them with Doctor Dean's garlic, and still they died. Even the fresh air on the verandah did nothing to save their lives.'

Her pleasures were those of any normal girl of her background and age. She and her colleagues visited the local cafés or went sometimes to tea-dances at the palais, where the competition was intense.

'Nottingham was packed with beautiful girls, some earning as much as two pounds a week at Player's. They could afford to bleach their hair and buy lipstick. None of us could, and anyway Matron would have frowned on both.'

Despite sincere efforts to feed the young nurses adequately, probationers who worked long hours were always hungry. Chips with everything was their standard diet, and happiness was a rich cream cake to finish the meal, and a bar of chocolate to take home to nibble in bed. Swollen ankles, chapped hands and a rumbling tummy were often the lot of the probationers, who were always short of cash. Unquestionably nurses at all levels were underpaid, and it was clear that all was not well in nursing in relation to educational training, salary and working conditions.

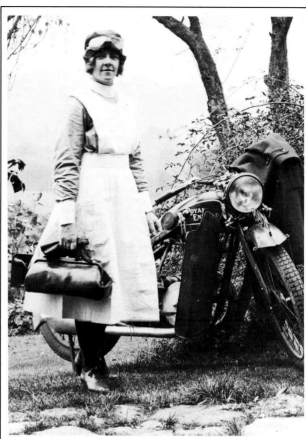

A district nurse of the early 1930s poses in front of her motor cycle—undoubtedly a great help in getting about in remote areas.

a trade union which would engage in collective bargaining, and even threatened strike action to improve pay and conditions of service. However, their view was not shared by the main body of nurses who, although they resented the penny-pinching attitude of hospital managements, were steeped in the traditions that had made nursing a vocation and regarded collective activity as a betrayal of the principles that had always motivated the lives of professional nurses.

The Athlone Committee

In 1937 the College of Nursing set up another committee, this time under Lord Athlone, which produced its first report in 1939, urgently advising that some mechanism be established to determine the pay and conditions of nurses. It also made a second, quite revolutionary recommendation that recognition should be given to a second grade of nurse to be known as 'assistant nurse'. As in the past, the report was widely circulated, but little useful action was taken.

Not unnaturally, existing conditions in the profession were hotly discussed in the 1920s and 1930s by the more militant elements among the nurses. They talked of forming

Preparations for war

In the mid-1930s nursing was not a popular choice for young women. Low pay and unacceptable working conditions were hardly likely to appeal to young recruits, and it was a matter of some concern to the government when, early in 1939, the Ministry of Health calculated the number of nurses who would be needed if war broke out.

The armed forces had asked for 5000 trained nurses, but it was estimated that between 34,000 and 67,000 would be needed to man the first-aid posts for the emergency hospitals designated to care for expected air-raid casualties. In all, there were only 60,000 trained nurses in Britain and it was

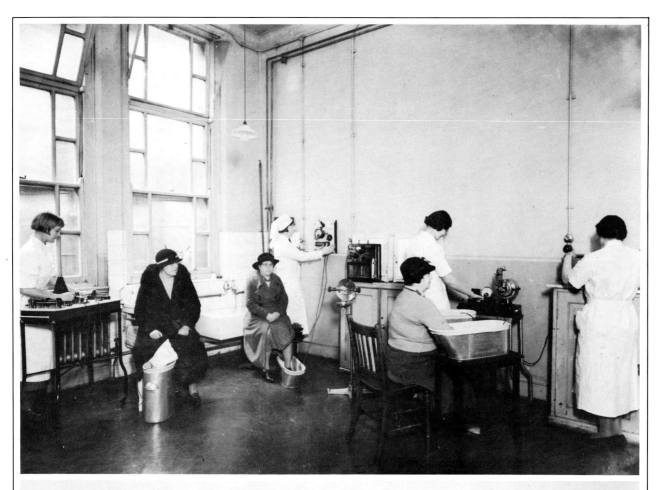

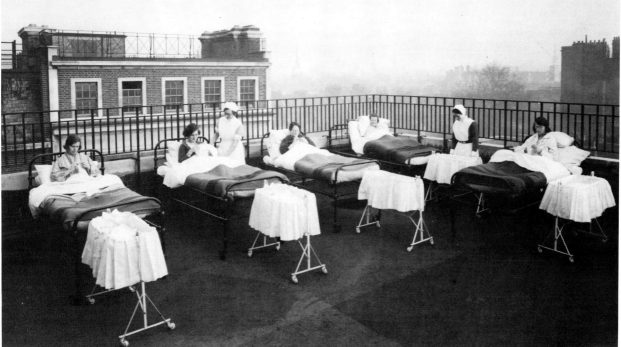

Top *Nurses giving electric therapeutic treatment to women outpatients at University College Hospital, London, c.1930.*
Above *A maternity unit with mothers, children and nurses enjoying fresh air on the roof of University College Hospital in the 1930s.*

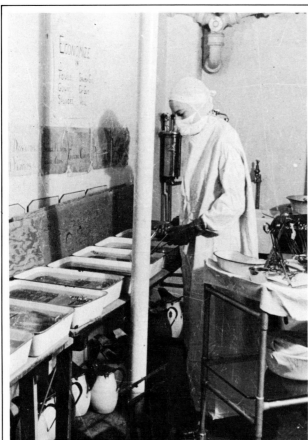

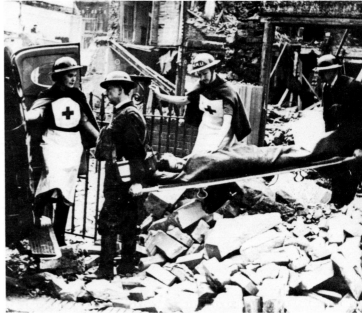

Above VADs help stretcher-bearers to remove a casualty after a bombing raid during the London Blitz.
Left The sister in charge of the operating theatre at Guy's Hospital, London, checks her equipment. Nightly German air raids kept the hospitals busy in 1940–41.
Opposite A nurse holding a baby inside its specially designed gas mask.
Below Blood donors provided an essential service in wartime Britain.

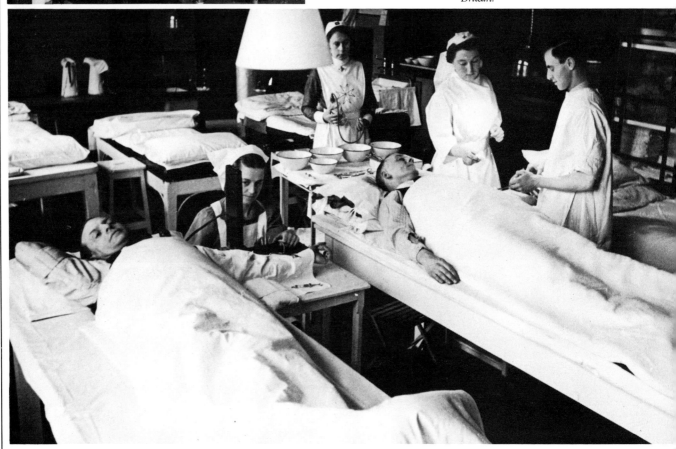

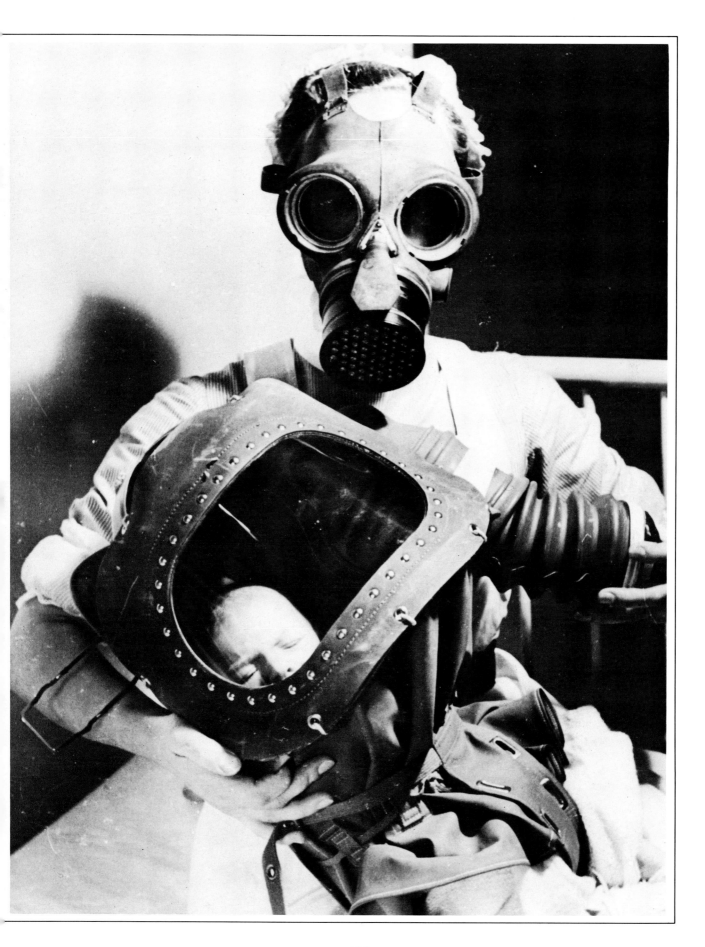

obvious that new recruits were urgently needed. A Civil Nursing Reserve was formed from women of all grades of training and experience, which gathered in some 7000 nurses and 3000 assistant nurses. In addition, an entirely new contingent of helpers – untrained volunteers called 'nursing auxiliaries' – was recruited. Thus, when war was declared another 20,000 nurses were available.

Just as the VADs had been unpopular with the trained nurses in the First World War, so now the members of the Civil Nursing Reserve irritated the highly disciplined personnel of the services with their own traditions and established hierarchy. The armed forces were also faced with problems over their unregistered nursing auxiliaries. Nurses of Queen Alexandra's Imperial Military Nursing Service had always been accorded officer status. Should this be extended to unregistered nurses? There were other matters, too, relating to officer privileges, such as first-class travel in uniform, board and lodging allowance and accommodation. Matters became so complicated that it was finally decided to withdraw 'officer' privileges from VAD nurses. This, much to their annoyance, meant exclusion from officers' clubs.

Nursing auxiliaries had 50 hours training before being allowed into the hospital wards, where they performed the normal domestic duties. Many of these VADs complained to their council, which in turn made it known to the War Office that 'many VAD members were people of high intelligence and capacity, and it was felt their gifts fitted them for something considerably better than mere routine and hard work.' As a result of this, an instruction was issued in 1940 relieving the VADs of all heavy domestic work, which was taken over by RAMC orderlies. At the same time it was clear that VADs were not qualified to take on full civilian nursing duties, a situation which again created problems in civilian hospitals where the VADs, having clearly defined and restricted duties, needed domestic back-up, which meant more personnel and higher costs.

Nursing in wartime

The Red Cross was not to be caught unprepared by the outbreak of war. Early in March 1939 it had been decided to overhaul the joint organization of the British Red Cross Society and the Order of St John. An emergency committee was formed. Contact was made with service departments and early in September the formal instrument setting up a war organization was sealed by the two bodies.

At the end of August a unit of VAD military members had slipped off to reinforce military hospitals in Egypt, and the mobilization orders despatched from the VAD council offices had resulted in every service hospital in the United Kingdom receiving its prescribed VAD quota. At the same time the members of the Civil Nursing Reserve were assembling at the emergency hospitals to which they had been posted, from the largest voluntary hospitals to the smallest

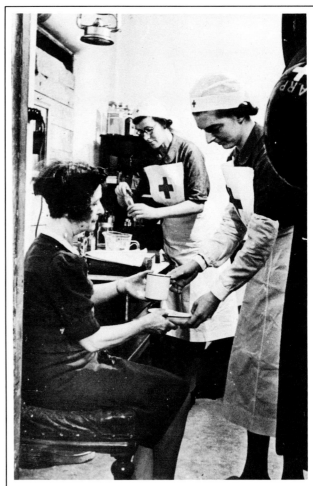

Nurses in a first aid post attached to an air raid shelter in Oxford Street, London, offer assistance to a casualty.

units administered by local authorities. Large mental institutions had been cleared of their inmates and hutted hospitals erected. Even the casual wards, a home-from-home for tramps, were made ready for use.

Many Red Cross and St John members had volunteered and had been trained for duty in civil defence first-aid posts. These existed at strategic points in London and in every town and city, and were manned around the clock. The Central Detachment Department was concerned with the staffing of ambulance trains which were kept in convenient sidings, their crews billeted close at hand, so that they could take the trains out at a moment's notice.

Yet in spite of all the precautions and preparations nobody was really prepared for what eventually happened. Nobody had imagined that this war, unlike those that had gone before, would be 'total' war, involving the massive aerial bombardment of cities teeming with civilians, and that it would put nurses from all the countries at war into the front line of battle.

As the theatres of war spread, so did the demand for nurses. They worked alongside the troops, sometimes under conditions which would have challenged Florence

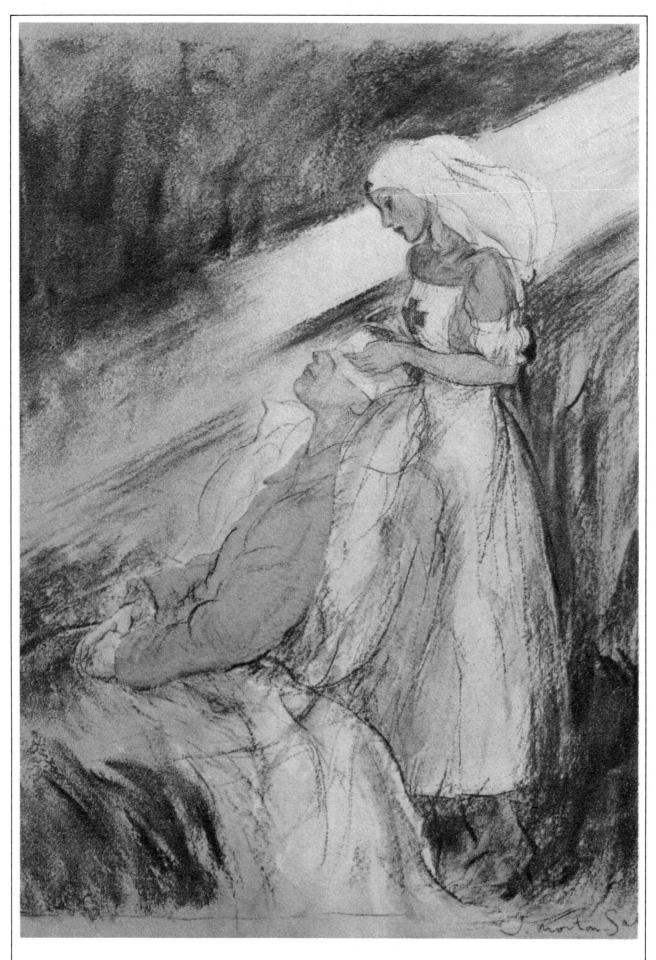

The Red Cross of Comfort by J. Morton Sale, a traditional view of the role of a nurse in wartime.

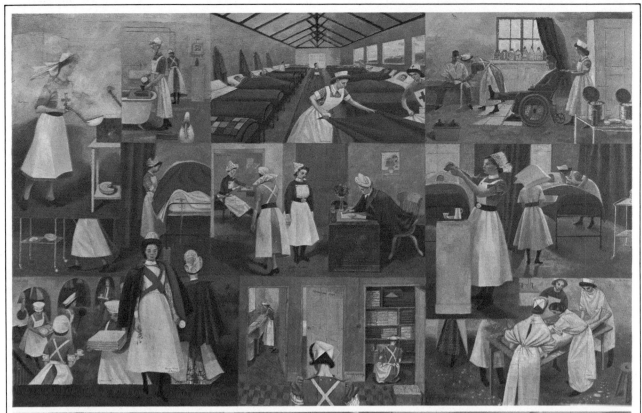

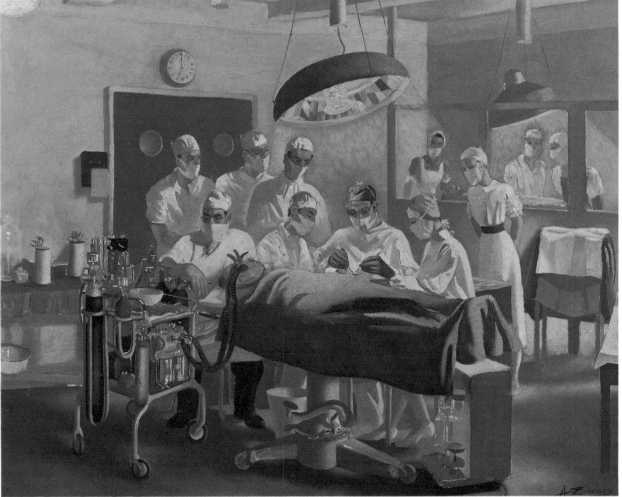

Top St Thomas' Hospital in Evacuation Quarters, *by Evelyn Dunbar, a vivid portrayal of the many and varied activities of a hospital in wartime.*

Above *The disfiguring injuries suffered by many airmen in the Second World War presented a special problem. Here Archibald McIndoe and his team of plastic surgeons are seen operating at the Queen Victoria Plastic and Jaw Injury Centre, East Grinstead. Painting by Anna Zinkeisen, 1944.*

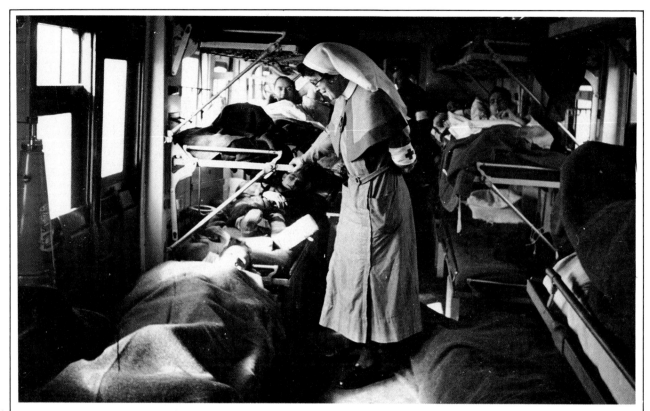

A hospital train in Britain carrying men wounded at the Battle of El Alamein, who are being taken to military hospitals.

Nightingale's ingenuity. Wearing battledress and often khaki trousers, their tin helmets firmly on their heads, they performed prodigies of valour. They served in every war zone and in every climate. Wherever the action was, there too were the nurses dealing with the wounded, smiling, patient and helpful. In the RAF they were trained to make parachute jumps. Some manned advance casualty stations. They kept calm when the hospital ships were torpedoed and some gave their lives to save those of their patients.

Nursing heroines

Nearly every war in history has produced unsung heroines. Among them were the nurses in England who carried on their day-to-day duties when the sky was dark with falling bombs, who gave first-aid to the wounded, who helped when babies were born in bomb-shelters, who comforted their terrified patients in hospitals and who stood firm when the operating theatres in which they were working were rocked by blast.

Edith Cavell was an inspiration to many nurses. One of them, Mary Lindell, joined the Red Cross in the First World War and nursed in French field hospitals. She married a Frenchman, the Comte de Milleville, had three children, and between the wars lived in Paris. In 1941 she was arrested

for helping Allied soldiers to escape and was sentenced to 11 years' imprisonment, a sentence she challenged. Her impudence so confounded the president of the court that he changed her sentence to one of nine months. The moment she was freed from prison, she made her way to England and became immediately involved in resistance work. Returning to France, she was arrested and sent to Ravensbruck concentration camp, which she survived. She later devoted herself to helping victims of Nazi persecution.

Helen Rodriguez, matron of a tiny hospital in Burma, found herself coping with 400 casualties after a Japanese air-raid. Since there was nobody else to take the initiative, she made herself responsible for the hospital and for its patients. Single-handed she defused a bomb and later successfully amputated a gangrenous leg, though she had never before seen such an operation.

She was awarded the George Medal for saving sick and badly wounded Indian soldiers abandoned in the shambles of the British retreat. The Japanese, who suspected her of being a spy, began interrogating her. She was saved by an interpreter who recognized her as being the matron of the hospital in which his sister had been nursed. Thereafter, in an internment camp, she organized and nursed the internees, seeing them through sickness and starvation and cruelties until they were liberated in 1945.

Andrée de Jongh, born in Brussels the year after Edith Cavell's execution there, was also inspired to follow her

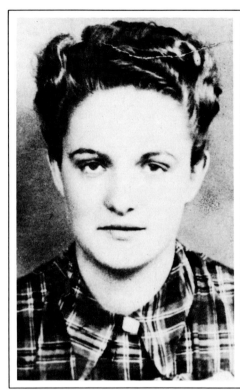

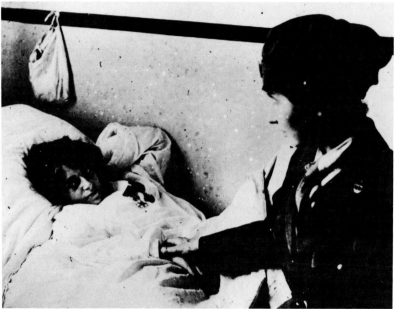

Above *Henriette Maud-Fraser, a nurse who was awarded the Légion d'Honneur and the Croix de Guerre for her work in France in the First World War.*
Left *Odette Malossane, a French nurse who played a gallant role in the resistance movement during the German occupation in the Second World War.*

example. She became a nurse, and worked with some of Cavell's nurses in her hospital. During the German occupation of Belgium in the Second World War she founded an escape route which ran for hundreds of miles from Brussels to Spain. As a result of her initiative many British air-crew shot down over France, Belgium and Holland were ferried back to England to continue the fight. After the War she went to Ethiopia, where she became matron of a leper hospital in Addis Ababa.

Another heroine was young Odette Malossane, who was matron of a small field hospital at Vassieux in the Vercors in France, which was filled mainly with members of the resistance movement. She was subsequently one of the nurses in the party of wounded soldiers (four of them Germans), doctors and civilians who, fleeing from the enemy, took refuge in a grotto in the Vercors region in July 1944. Without food and with only the moisture dripping from stalactites in the grotto to drink, doctors and nurses did all they could for the casualties under their care.

On 27 July the Germans burst into the cave and, at gunpoint, ordered everyone out. The prisoners were separated into two groups. The stretcher cases, despite the pleas of the wounded German soldiers, were immediately massacred. The rest were herded into lorries and sent to various destinations. Later, the nurses, including Odette Malossane, were sent to concentration camps, where they died.

More recently, in 1984, after the Falklands War, yet another young nurse displayed the heroism and dedication to duty which earned her the title of 'Angel of the Falklands'. Barbara Chick, aged 35, was one of the eight victims of the fire which destroyed the King Edward Memorial Hospital in Stanley. Defying orders to abandon rescue attempts, she saved four patients, but was overcome by smoke and fumes while entering the hospital for the fifth time.

Nursing medals

In Nov. 1984 an unusual sale took place in London, at which Sotheby and Co. auctioned 'Orders, Medals and Decorations', including a collection of nursing awards formed by Captain K. J. Douglas-Morris, a retired naval officer.

Among these medals was an important pair for the Zulu War, comprising the Royal Red Cross and the campaign medal for the war in South Africa 1877-9. The former was presented by Queen Victoria at Windsor to Mrs J. C. Deeble, Superintendent of Nurses.

In 1879 Mrs Deeble had been ordered to South Africa to take charge of the nursing staff, and was subsequently reported for her conspicuously good service and thanked by command of the queen. Mrs Deeble's Royal Red Cross was the tenth to be awarded. Of the previous nine issued, eight had been bestowed on ladies with royal connections and the other on Florence Nightingale. Mrs Deeble's must therefore be considered the second awarded to a woman for nursing services.

An exceptional group were the medals awarded to Nursing Sister Mary Jerrard, Army Medical Department and Military Nursing Establishment, comprising the Royal Red Cross, Victoria, and the campaign medals for South Africa,

1877, without clasp, Egypt, 1882, 1 clasp, The Nile 1884–5, and Khedive's Star, dated 1884–6.

Mary Jerrard was attached to the Army Medical Department during the Zulu War of 1877–9, and during the Egyptian campaign saw service with the military nursing establishment. She had been posted to Wadi Halfa by local general order on 15 Sept. 1884, and thus took part in the Nile operations of that year.

A very rare medal indeed, of which only nine were awarded to nurses, was given to Sister Gertrude Ireland for her services and those of her colleagues in the Hong Kong plague of 1894. In May of that year an outbreak of bubonic plague of epidemic proportions descended on the inhabitants of Hong Kong, and by September over 2000 people had died from its ravages. The matron, Sister Gertrude Ireland, and other nurses trained in London hospitals, all volunteered to serve in the government plague hospitals as well as continuing their duties in the government hospital.

The Colonial Surgeon, Doctor L. C. B. Eyres, had nothing but praise for the dedicated work of the nurses. In his submission he wrote:

> It is most difficult to describe the horrors of the work the Sisters undertook, they had the risk of infection from a disease at that time little known, but whose terrors are historical. The majority of their patients on admission being in a state of furious delirium, needing constant attention and causing the most distressing scenes. They (the nurses) had to serve for long consecutive hours in wards where the heat of the atmosphere, in spite of the finest ventilation that could be given, was most oppressive, amid odours of the most offensive description from the involuntary exertions of the patients they had to clean. *Extract from Sotheby's Catalogue, Nov. 1984.*

Sister Mary Foley, QAIMNS, saw service in France and Belgium from Aug. 1914 until Nov. 1918. She was awarded several medals, one of which was the Military Medal, given her 'for coolness and gallantry displayed in the performance of her duties when a casualty station was heavily shelled'. Sister Foley was in fact twice mentioned in despatches, and also received the OBE, RRC 1914 Star and Victory Medal.

Some rare civil gallantry awards were also made to nurses, and one, an Albert Medal (2nd Class, in bronze), was presented to Nurse Florence Alice Allen 'for gallantry in saving life at Quetta in 1935'. During the Baluchistan earthquake at Quetta, on 31 May 1935, 'at the risk of her own life and at the cost of terrible injuries to her leg, Nurse Allen saved the life of a child in her charge by throwing herself across the cot.' Her injuries were so serious that it was a long time before she was well enough to receive her award, which was eventually made by King Edward VIII.

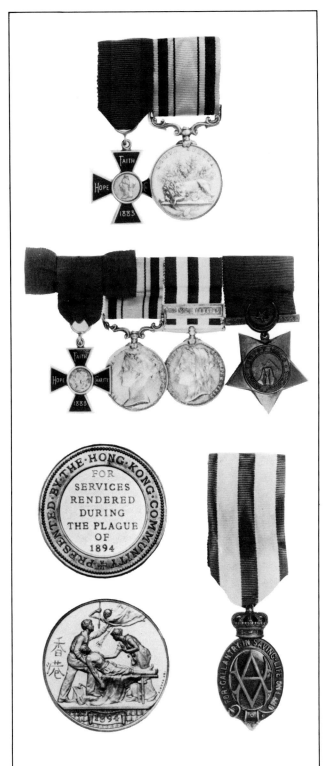

Top *The Royal Red Cross and the campaign medal given to Mrs J. C. Deeble.*
Centre *The group of four medals awarded to Sister Mary Jerrard for her services in South Africa and Egypt.*
Above left *The obverse and reverse of the medal presented to nurses for their work during the Hong Kong plague of 1894.*
Above right *The Albert Medal awarded to Nurse Florence Alice Allen.*

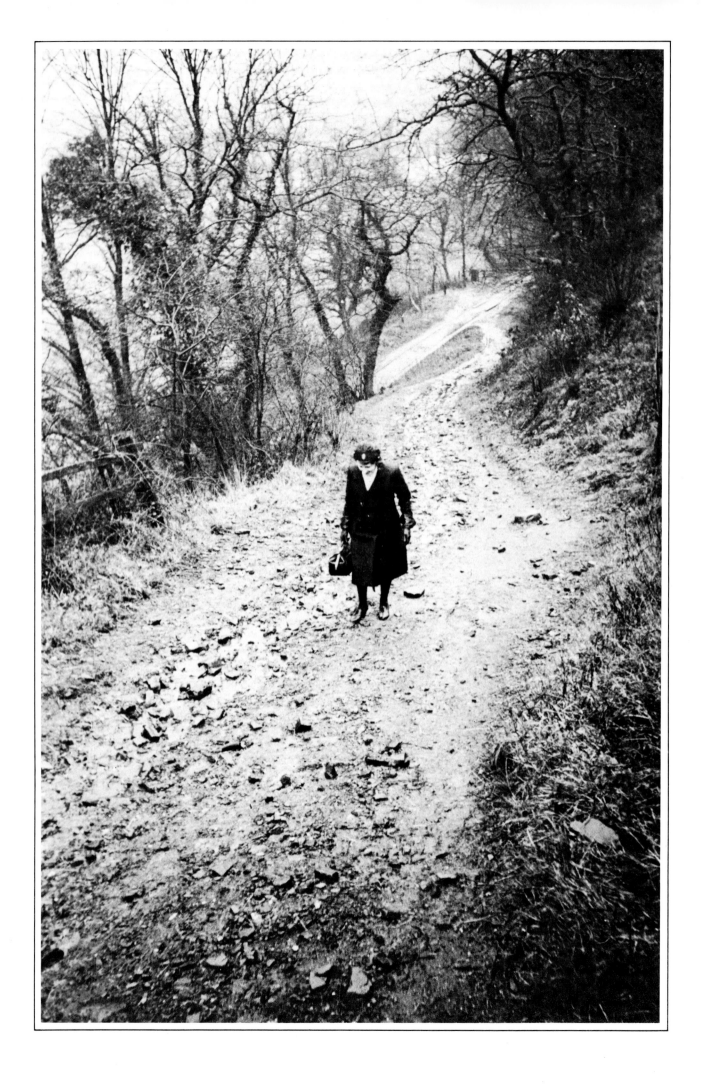

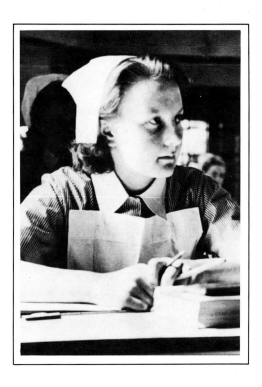

Postwar developments

'Nothing,' wrote J. B. Priestley in 1940 in his *Postscripts* (published by Heinemann), 'has impressed me more in this bombing battle of London than the continued high courage and resolution, not only of the wives and mothers, but also of the crowds of nurses, secretaries, clerks, telephone girls, shop assistants, waitresses, who, morning after morning have turned up for duty, neat as ever – rather pink about the eyes perhaps, and smiling rather tremulously, but still smiling.'

Women had at last come into their own. They had proved that, like London during the Blitz, 'they could take it,' and they tried, under morale-shattering circumstances, to carry on as usual.

As with most other organizations under constant threat, the work of the office of the Royal College of Nursing was made increasingly difficult by shortage of staff, though those who were left laboured twice as long and twice as hard, and the various negotiations to better the lot of nurses, begun before the war, continued on their laborious and labyrinthine peregrinations.

Top *Student nurses attending a lecture. Advances in medical knowledge meant that nurses' training had to be adapted to meet new needs.*
Opposite *A district nurse in wartime Britain. In country areas her work inevitably involved covering large distances on foot.*

In 1938 the Athlone Committee, as mentioned in the previous chapter, had recommended the setting up of a 'nurses' salary committee', and in 1943 such a committee was established under the chairmanship of Lord Rushcliffe. The committee was composed of representatives of employers and of nursing bodies, and was one of the first organizations to consider the salaries and conditions of nurses on a national basis. At this time there was a tremendous shortfall in the number of nurses available. The armed forces had absorbed large numbers of them, most of whom preferred to work in the services rather than with the sick in civilian hospitals.

The Second World War blazed new trails in medicine and surgery and, consequently, in nursing techniques. The discovery and use of antibiotics, such as penicillin, revolutionized the treatment of virulent infections, and new drugs and new methods of treatment hastened the recovery of patients, and got them out of bed much more quickly than had happened in the past.

In the First World War facial injuries had been given a low priority, and the resultant mortality of soldiers and airmen from shock and lack of treatment had been high. In the Second World War great importance was given to the plastic surgery units known, flippantly, as 'Max Factor' (Maxillo-Facial) Units. These were small mobile units which dealt entirely with facial injuries. The role of the nurses who were working in these units was to clean up the worst of the injuries sustained by the burnt or injured men in order to produce a healthy canvas for the reconstructive surgery

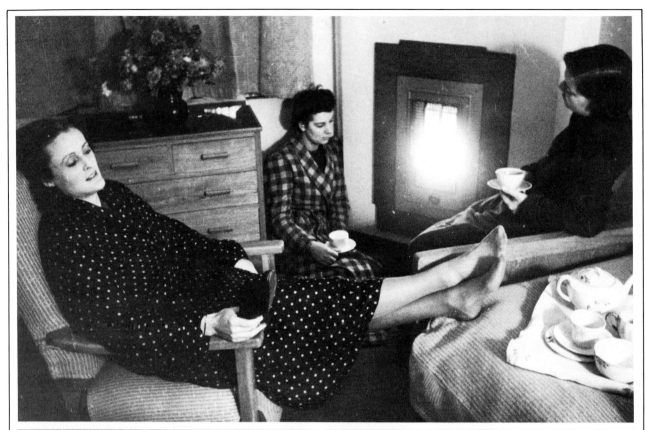

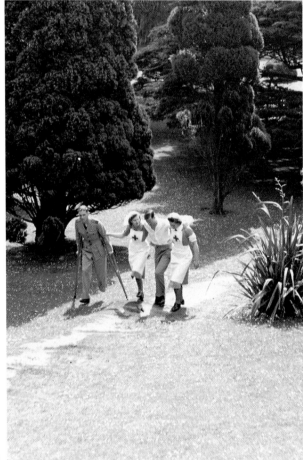

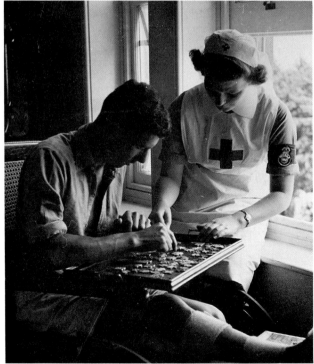

Top Nurses at Westminster Hospital in wartime take an
opportunity to put their feet up.
Above A VAD nurse helps an injured airman undergoing
rehabilitation to complete a jigsaw puzzle.
Left Nurses walking in the grounds of a hospital with airmen
who have suffered limb damage.

which would take place later in hospitals at Park Prewitt, Bangor, and the Queen Victoria Hospital at East Grinstead, Sussex.

The work, carried on in what had originally been a small cottage-hospital, was to become famous throughout the world, for it was here that Archibald McIndoe and his team of plastic surgeons made medical history. To Ward 3 came airmen burned and mutilated in enemy and allied aircraft. Their restoration in mind and body and the founding of their unique Guinea Pig Club aroused universal admiration. There was only one way of being admitted to its exclusive membership – through excruciating pain – for it was restricted to aircraft blaze survivors only. It was said at the time that there were only four ways in which men could be admitted to Ward 3 for treatment – 'mashed, boiled, fried or roasted'. At the end of the war there were 644 members of the Guinea Pig Club, some of whom had undergone as many as 80 operations.

The National Health Service

Meanwhile, in the background, changes that would affect not only the general public but eventually the whole of the nursing profession were in the melting pot. On 1 Dec. 1942 the famous *Beveridge Report* was made public. The document ran to 100,000 words and contained 23 proposals. It sought to effect a complete postwar reconstruction of the social services and its chief recommendations included unemployment insurance for all, free medical and hospital treatment, child benefits, and marriage and death grants.

A debate in Parliament in 1943 showed that the government accepted in principle the institution of children's allowances, a comprehensive medical service, and the universality of benefits and funeral grants, but maintained reservations about the financial implications.

A widening of the national health scheme was the inevitable outcome of the extension of social policy in matters of health. Official discussions began in 1943, and early in the following year appeared the government's white paper, *A National Health Service*, which aimed at preparing 'a comprehensive cover for health provided for all people alike'. What it proposed was a complete service, available to everyone who wished to make use of it and covering all forms of medical care. The white paper was, however, very carefully worded so as to allow the continuance of private practice.

The hospital service, severely tested by the war and found wanting in many ways, was to be redeveloped by co-operation between local authorities working together in joint bodies, which would have the task of framing, together with the medical profession, 'area plans for securing complete health services in their several areas'. The voluntary hospitals would be brought into the plan and would participate as autonomous agencies.

The application of this revolutionary scheme was to prove

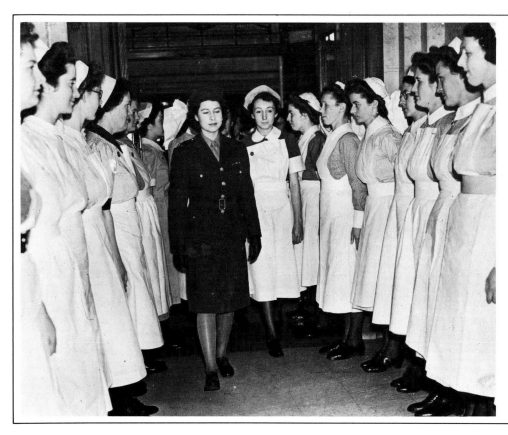

Princess (later Queen) Elizabeth inspects a line of nurses while paying a visit to the Royal College of Nursing in July 1945.

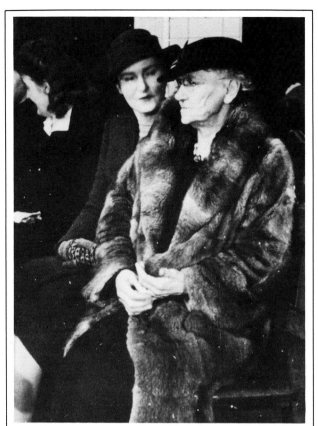

The mother and sister of Aneurin Bevan, the minister of health in the postwar Labour government, take their turn in a health centre waiting room.

a very complex matter, involving local authorities in every part of the country and voluntary hospitals of every size and grade of efficiency. It fell to Aneurin Bevan, as minister of health, to frame the final proposals, which became law in Nov. 1946.

The principal change made was that the service was to be organized on a functional, not a regional basis. Thus hospital autonomy was to disappear, and all hospitals, local authority and voluntary alike, were to be merged in regional hospital boards, centred on the country's medical schools, but the teaching hospitals themselves were to remain independent. Although they were to lose their hospitals the local authorities were to develop other health services, especially the preventive ones, and to ensure close collaboration with the hospital boards.

From the nursing point of view, the white paper was a bitter disappointment. Importance was given to the provision of complete domiciliary service, but there was hardly any recognition of the fact that the success of public health hospital and clinical hospital alike depended entirely on an adequate supply of well-trained nurses.

The Royal College of Nursing drew up a draft memorandum on a *Plan of Nursing in a National Health Service*, which formed the basis of discussion at the annual conference that year. The conference stressed the need to develop all branches of nursing in relation to the National Health Service from a base of general and professional education.

It dealt with the importance of expanding the domiciliary nursing service to include, where possible, a full-time, as well as a visiting service. Health centres were proposed, with more comprehensive functions than the grouped medical practices outlined in the white paper. Schemes were drafted for co-ordinating public health and institutional nursing policy within each local government area, and for improving in other ways the preventive and curative health service which was assumed to be the right of every citizen.

The Whitley Council

Under the terms of the National Health Service Act the minister of health was empowered to determine the machinery for negotiating pay and conditions for all NHS employees, but health departments, which assisted grant-aided hospitals, could apply pressure. The minister decided to adopt the Whitley Council system, which had been used in the Civil Service since 1920, to negotiate pay and conditions of work within the hospital service. One functional Whitley Council was to be wholly concerned with nurses and midwives.

The outcome of the first round of negotiations was to change the basis on which nurses were paid. Traditionally, hospital nurses had received a net salary and were provided with free board and lodging. The Whitley agreement introduced gross salaries, and nurses were then required to pay for their board and lodgings at rates laid down nationally. The resultant 'cash in hand' was niggardly.

In 1948, following representation from the Royal College of Nursing, the post of chief nursing officer was created at the Ministry of Health, and this officer, among other duties, had responsibility for advising the minister of health on all matters connected with nursing. The first chief nursing officer was Dame Katherine Watt, formerly matron-in-chief of the Princess Mary Royal Air Force Nursing Service.

On a lighter note, it was in 1944 that the Royal College of Nursing had applied for its grant of arms. The College submitted designs to the College of Arms for a coat of arms. The first reaction of the College was as follows. 'You cannot,' they said, 'carry your arms on a shield, since you are a women's organization, you may only carry your arms on a lozenge.' In 1946, after repeated representations, the College of Arms finally conceded that the Royal College of Nursing might carry its arms on a shield because of the distinguished part nurses had played in the Second World War, working, as they had done, close to the front lines.

Emblazoned on a blue shield are the sun and the stars denoting the day and night service nurses give. The shield is surmounted by an open book of learning and by a Roman lamp authorized by the College of Arms as the heraldic

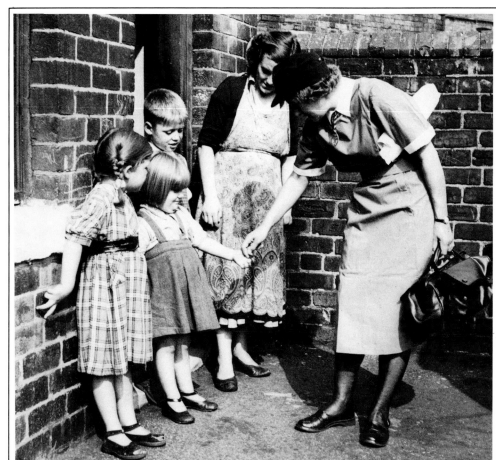

Left *A district nurse on her round of visits greets a small child.*
Below *A nurse provides medicine for a sick child. Efficient home nursing in the postwar years was responsible for much of the improvement in the nation's health.*

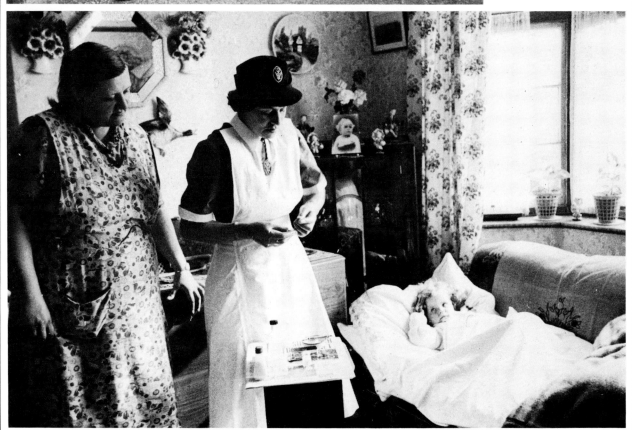

symbol of nursing. Inscribed at the base of the shield is the motto *Tradimus Lampada* ('We hand on the torch').

In 1947 Ethel Bedford Fenwick died at the age of 90. Tributes to her poured in from all over the world, and the indomitable lady would have been much gratified to read the homage paid by the *British Journal of Nursing*, who wrote of her 'as the greatest nurse within living memory'. Her death brought to an end an important era in the history of nursing, to which she had contributed far more than she had ever been given credit for. No official honour was ever awarded her, but she must have gained great satisfaction from the knowledge that she was State Registered Nurse No. 1.

Towards a new structure

In the early 1950s a standing nursing advisory committee was set up, once again to advise ministers on nursing matters. This was the first machinery at government level in which nurses had a distinct advisory role, for a matter of deep concern at the time was the lack of influence of nurses on hospital authorities. The matron of a hospital did not normally have right of attendance at meetings of the hospital authority. As a result others, unqualified in this particular, tended to speak on behalf of the nurses.

The profession was also increasingly concerned about the lack of recognition for hospital matrons, and it was becoming more difficult to get candidates to fill the post of matron and assistant matron because of this problem.

Under the chairmanship of Brian Salmon a government committee was set up in 1963 'To advise on the senior nursing staff structure in the hospital service (Ward Sister and above), the administrative functions of the respective grades and the methods of preparing staff to occupy them.' The committee recommended a management structure which incorporated three levels – first line, middle and top, two grades being identified at each level. The pinnacle of the structure was the grade of chief nursing officer – responsible to the hospital authority, whose meetings she would attend. It also recommended management training to prepare for the posts at each level.

The committee's recommendations were accepted by the Ministry of Health and implementation began in 1969. The

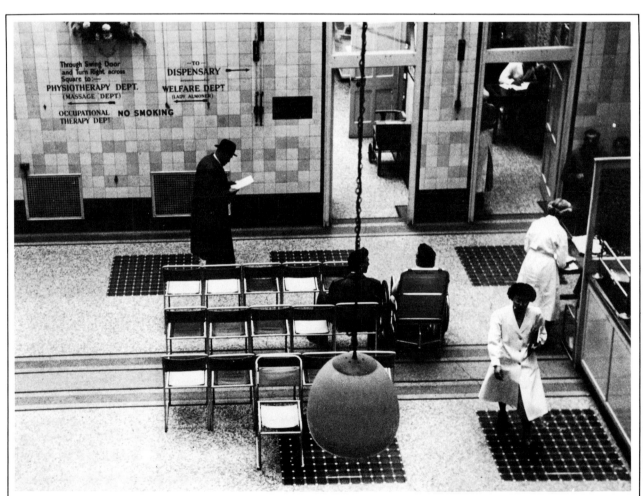

The out-patients' department at St Bartholomew's Hospital, London, in the early 1950s, a few years after the founding of the National Health Service.

new management structures attracted considerable opposition from the medical profession, which considered that the emphasis being placed on management denigrated the importance of clinical practice and undermined the role of the ward sister. The new 'nursing officer' titles received adverse comment and the discontinuation of 'matron' as a recognized title was particularly criticized, despite the fact that men were moving into positions which would formerly have carried this title.

A further committee on nursing was set up in 1970 under the chairmanship of Professor Asa Briggs to review the role of the nurse and midwife in the hospital and the community, and the education and training required for that role, so that the best use should be made of available manpower to meet the future needs of an integrated health service. This wide-ranging study, supported by research, made far-reaching recommendations concerning all aspects of nursing. Unfortunately, the only significant action to date resulting from the recommendations was the establishment in 1980, within one statutory structure, of the regulations relating to the nursing, midwifery and health-visiting professions. The five new statutory bodies established, one at United Kingdom level and one in each country within the United Kingdom, together assumed the functions of the nine statutory and training bodies which had previously carried responsibility in this particular sphere. The United Kingdom Central Council for Nursing, Midwifery and Health Visiting maintains the professional register of all nurses, midwives and health visitors in the country. It develops standards of education and training, establishes and improves standards of professional conduct, and protects the public from unsafe practitioners.

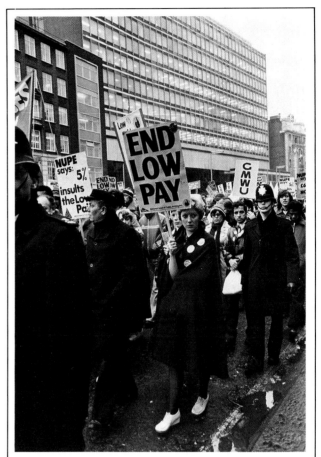

Nurses taking part in a demonstration by public service employees. The rising tide of inflation in the late 1970s led to increasing militancy amongst lower-paid workers.

Further changes

In 1974 the National Health Service was reorganized, bringing within one administrative structure the hospital services and the personal health services previously provided by local health authorities. Health authorities responsible for the provision of health services within a defined area were set up and a nursing officer was one of the team of chief officers at health authority level.

The reorganization of the senior nursing staff structure which had resulted from the Salmon Committee recommendations (and a similar reorganization of the nursing management structures of the local authority nursing services which had resulted from the recommendations of the Mayston Committee) meant that those who had held posts as chief nursing officer were equipped to fulfil the new roles at health authority level. This strengthened the position of the profession in pressing for, and achieving, recognition of the nurse as a full and equal member of the team of officers at both area and district level within the reorganized health service.

In 1974 the Royal College of Nursing submitted evidence to the secretary of state for health and social services on *The State of Nursing 1974*. This highlighted many areas of concern relating to standards of care, staffing, education and training, and levels of pay. Inadequate pay had resulted from the rapid rise in the cost of living since 1974, and the College called for an independent enquiry into nurses' pay.

A committee of inquiry set up in 1974 under the chairmanship of Lord Halsbury made far-reaching recommendations. The overall increase in pay was to be in the region of 30%, the actual increase ranging as between grades, but the next few years were a time when government pay policies prevailed and inhibited increases in pay, particularly in the public sector.

In 1980, after a submission to the government for improvements in nurses' pay in the previous year, this vexed subject was referred to the Clegg Commission. The resultant increases were in the region of an overall 22%, but did not re-establish pay at the same comparable level as had been achieved in 1974. The report was not at all well received by the profession.

In 1981–2 the Nurses' and Midwives' Whitley Council made further submissions to the government for special

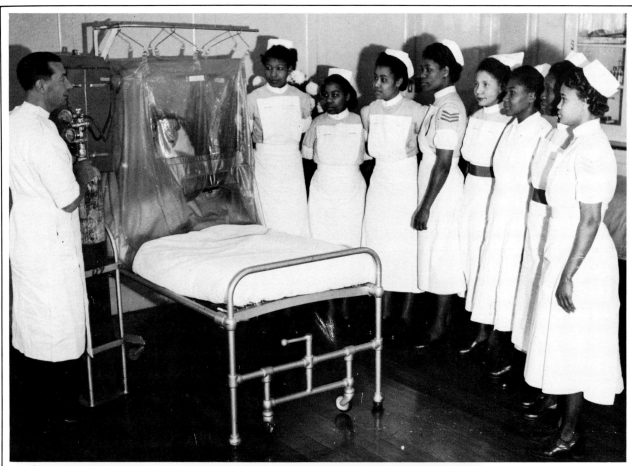

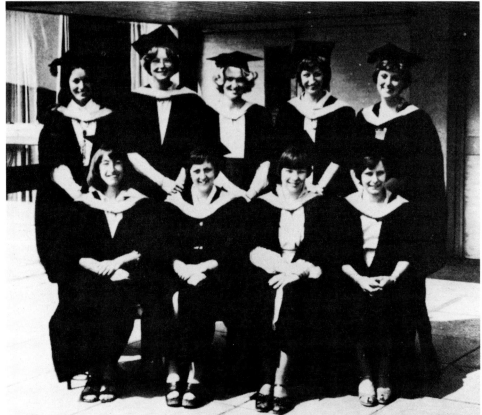

Above *Nurses from the West Indies in training at Hackney Hospital, London. In postwar Britain a general shortage of nurses led to a determined overseas recruitment campaign.*
Left *Graduate nurses at the Welsh School of Medicine in the mid-1970s. In the past few decades advances in medicine have led to a demand for more highly qualified nursing staff.*

treatment for nurses. The 1982 negotiations were protracted, some nurses engaged in industrial action and feelings ran high within the profession. The Royal College of Nursing, while applying pressure in all constitutional ways, maintained its traditional position of opposition to industrial action by nurses, and its members did not engage in such action. This was a major factor in attracting respect and support and in achieving an end to the dispute. The outcome was in fact an improved pay offer to cover a period of two years, but, more significantly, the government agreed to remove nurses' pay from the negotiating arena, and to establish an independent pay review for nurses and midwives. This body came into being in 1983.

The history of nurses' pay reflects little glory on successive governments which have either avoided the issue or temporized, for nurses' emoluments have never been maintained at an equitable level. On the occasions when significant improvements have been achieved, their value has been rapidly eroded by periods of escalation in the cost of living.

Educational developments

It is doubtful whether Florence Nightingale would have applauded the educational developments in nursing which took place in the late 1960s.

When the University of Edinburgh, through its Department of Nursing Studies, introduced an undergraduate programme to prepare students for registration as nurses and for a degree in an established discipline, other universities and, later, polytechnics followed their lead, the University of Manchester being the first to offer a degree in nursing. However, only a very small proportion of nurses in the United Kingdom are prepared for registration through undergraduate programmes.

Certain universities now offer higher degrees in nursing and a growing number of nurses study for degrees after qualifying as a nurse, a development facilitated by Open University studies. Some candidates possess a degree before embarking on nurse training. There are now chairs of nursing in five universities in the United Kingdom and one chair of nursing education. In short, nursing has achieved recognition as an academic discipline.

It is also interesting to note how much research in nursing has developed over the past 30 years. In 1972 the Committee on Nursing stated that it should become a research-based profession. However, nursing still remains largely 'unresearched', and there is need for increasing recognition of the importance of research in promoting improved standards of practice.

In 1977 the Royal College of Nursing became registered as a trade union. The spate of industrial relations legislation made it necessary for the College to acquire the rights and privileges of a trade union in order to continue effectively its

work in the negotiation of salaries and conditions for nurses and in the protection of its members as employees.

The change in membership requirements between 1960 and 1970 also meant that in that period the College had evolved from an elitist body into a comprehensive and fully representative professional one, admitting to membership all those holding a statutory nursing qualification or else in training for such a qualification.

The extent to which the development of the College as an organization has won respect and support from the nursing profession at large is reflected in its growth in membership from some 30,000 in the mid-1950s to more than 230,000 in 1984.

Changes in the National Health Service

In 1982 the National Health Service was restructured. This involved the dissolution of area health authorities and the establishment of district health authorities, so decreasing the size of the population for which an authority was responsible. It also involved a reorganization within the districts to create a structure which was more clinically orientated and more responsive to patient/client needs. Within the new structure the chief nurse retained her position as an equal member of the team of officers responsible to the health authority for the management of the totality of the nursing and midwifery services it provided.

In 1982 the secretary of state for social services set up a management enquiry into the NHS. The main recommendation related to the creation of a management board at health department level, and of general manager posts at health authority level and also at unit level within the internal structure of the individual health authorities. The recommendations were accepted for implementation, despite forceful expressions of concern by the major health care professions.

Their reservations were based on the general manager concept which involves those officers in overall control of the services provided by the health authority. For it is evident that the general manager will be the authorities' chief executive officer. The immediate effect on the nursing profession is that the chief nurse at authority level will not be ultimately responsible for the management of the authorities' nursing services. Her role, therefore, will become essentially an advisory one.

However, the profession, in particular through the Royal College of Nursing, has exerted strong pressure to ensure that the nurse still retains her responsibility for professional standards and for professional development. In addition, it has endeavoured to ensure that nurses at unit level remain professionally accountable to the chief nurse, although they will have a managerial accountability to the unit general managers. Moreover, nurses are eligible to apply for general manager posts.

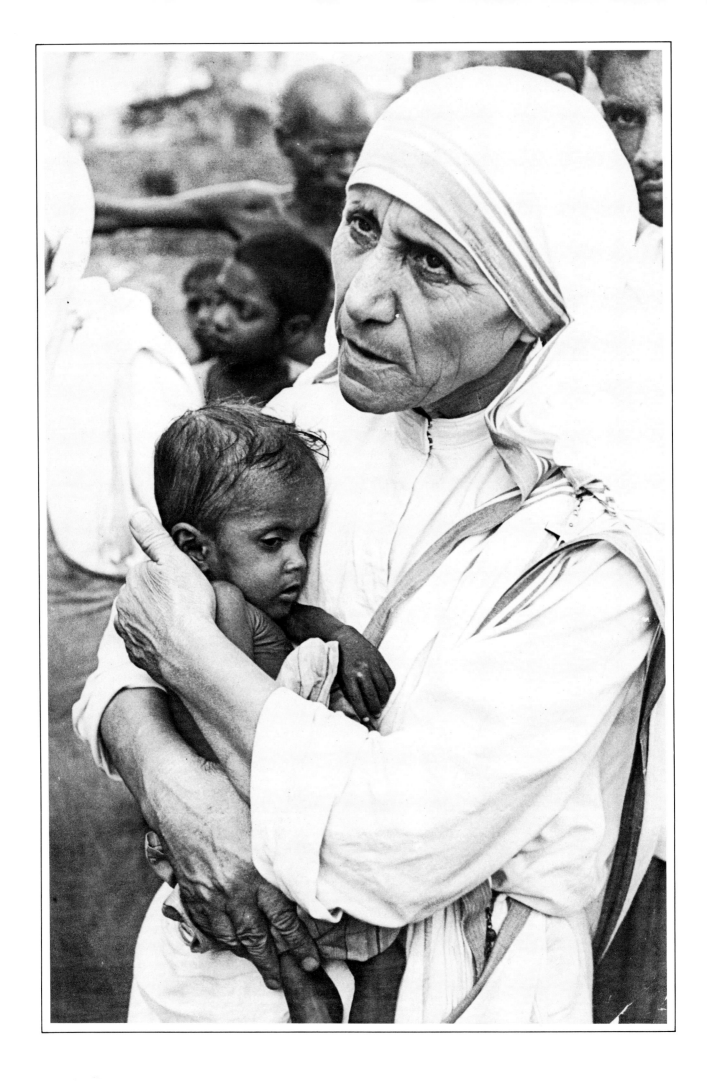

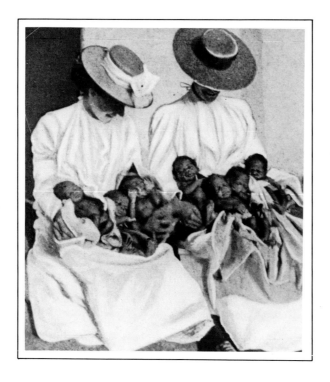

Nursing in the field

Nursing in the Third World

There is no doubt that Britain was the cradle of professional nursing, and that Florence Nightingale's hand-picked lady-nurses blazed pioneer trails throughout the world. Many countries built their nursing services on the principles laid down by Florence Nightingale. Today, of course, most countries have their own traditions and high professional standards which have made enormous contributions to the sum total of nursing knowledge and care.

Each country has its own methods and its own organizations for dealing with national disasters, which are backed up by the services of the great international relief organizations such as the Red Cross and Oxfam, who send out contingents of doctors and nurses with medicine, food, blankets and shelters for the stricken.

There are also many other organizations whose work is concerned with nursing in the field. Such a one is the Save the Children Fund, which operates world-wide. One of their trained nurses, Diana Lacey, having spent a year in a French-speaking Swiss hospital, returned to England to begin her midwifery training, in which she qualified in 1980. Instead of taking up a job in an Oxford hospital, she responded to an appeal by the Save the Children Fund for nurses to work in

Karamoja in northeastern Uganda, whose population was being decimated by famine. She later wrote:

'When we arrived we found skeletons along the rough roads. We were the first nurses in the area, and despite all our care and attention, ten to fifteen children died in our centre each day. Because of the high security risks we couldn't care for our charges during the hours of darkness. Imagine watching a child die because he is too weak to swallow the food we spoon into his mouth. Ten-year-olds weighed only three to four kilos, and once on the road to recovery each child was obsessed by the thought that food supplies might run out.

Our first port of call was Abim in Western Karamoja where another nurse and myself were the only two European nurses within a radius of three hundred miles. We had no radio communication, and for the first six weeks no form of transport, so we had to walk each day from our lodgings to the feeding unit.

Daily we fed and cared for five hundred children from tiny babies to twelve-year-olds. Each child had four feeds a day, which involved an endless round of preparation, distribution and supervision. Discipline was one of our main problems, after those posed by the endemic diseases which were rife.

Anaemia, a certain killer in the Third World, aggravated by severe malnutrition, posed an enormous problem, as it was difficult to find any adult healthy enough to give blood to a child.

Top *Nurses holding an armful of babies at a missionary hospital in Uganda in 1900.*
Opposite *Mother Teresa with a small child. Her nursing work in the Calcutta slums has won the admiration of the world.*

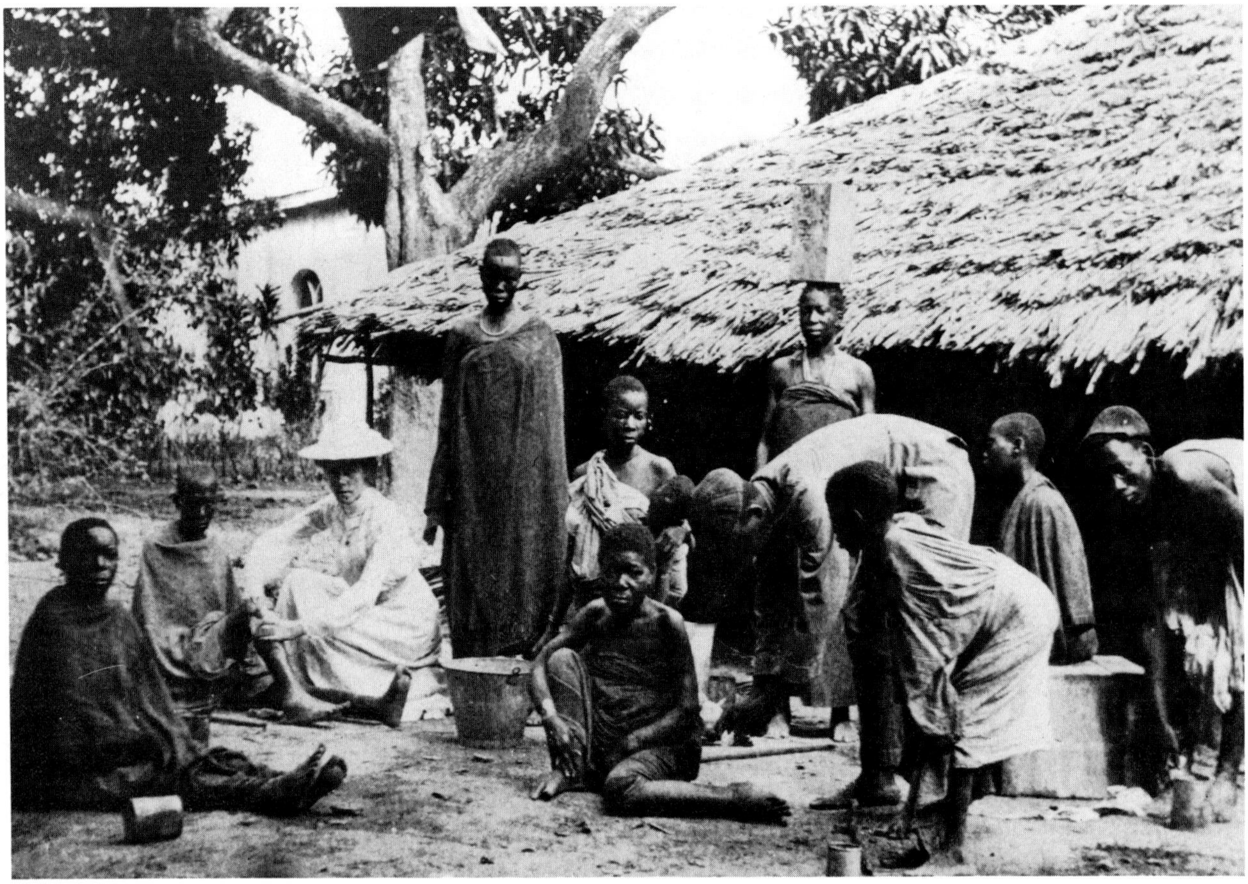

Patients at Rabai Hospital, Kenya, at the beginning of the century, one of whom is having a knee bandaged by a white nurse.

Some food was trucked in from Mombasa and some flown in, but, as everyone was starving, a thriving black market was soon in operation.'

One of her major tasks was to vaccinate the children against measles, one of the principal causes of death in the Third World. This again presented a great problem, for it was no easy matter to maintain a cold chain to keep the vaccine at the right temperature.

In 1956 three plastic surgeons, Sir Archibald McIndoe, and two of his pupils, Michael Wood and Thomas Rees, had conceived the idea of the African Medical and Research Foundation. The concept was an ambitious one – to provide a voluntary organization which would not only supplement the inadequate medical services of East Africa, but also concern itself with the initiation and assistance of field research in the area.

The area chosen was vast, covering Kenya, Tanganyika and Uganda. Here about 22 million people lived in an area the size of Western Europe. The ratio of doctors to patients was one to 30,000. The governments were desperately poor, so it was evident that the Foundation would have to be supported by voluntary contributions from Europe and the United States.

The first step was to initiate a flying doctor service which, since 1967, has flown more than five million miles, treated nearly 970,000 people, administered 1.2 million immunizations, performed 22,000 major operations, evacuated over 3000 emergency patients and carried out important programmes and projects, most of which involve nurses, both European and African.

At the beginning of 1983 two of AMREF's nurses, Sisters Sandcock and Robinson, were invited by the Uganda government to help Oxfam and Save the Children Fund to carry out the mass immunization programme desperately needed in Uganda. By the end of 1983 over 2 million vaccinations had been given to a population of 400,000 in the Arua region in northwestern Uganda. These were mainly against polio and measles. The teams also helped in setting up static immunization clinics as well as meeting with staff of local hospitals, dispensaries, clinics and other health centres.

Another group of young, dedicated French doctors and nurses, belonging to an organization known as Médecine du Monde, pledged themselves to bring medical and humanitarian aid to the embattled Afghans. Half the population has intestinal parasites, and nearly everyone suffers from malnutrition and from a chronic vitamin deficiency. The

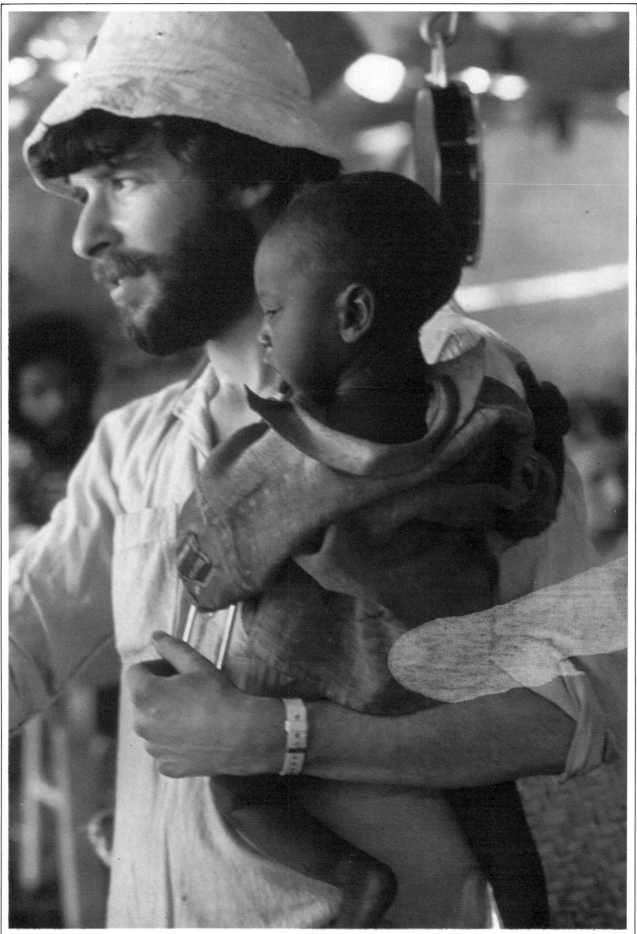

A Save the Children Fund nurse with a child at a refugee camp in the Sudan.

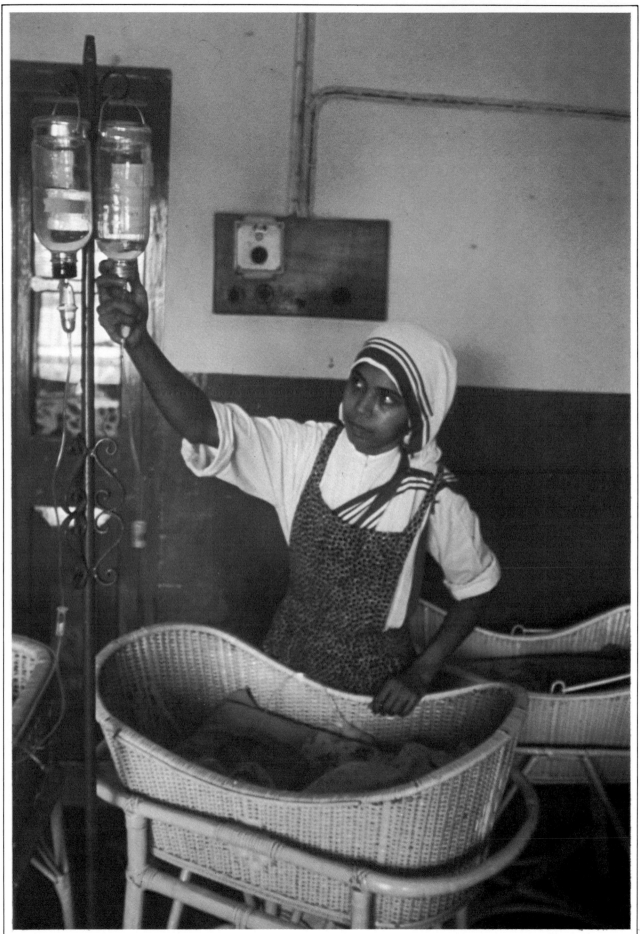

A nurse at work in a children's ward at Mother Teresa's hospital in Calcutta.

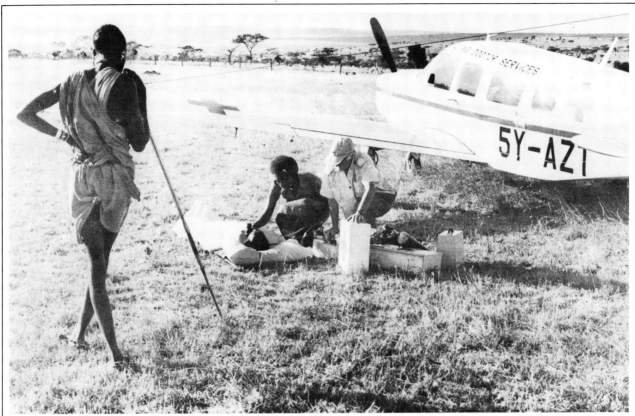

A patient in a remote part of Kenya receives emergency medical attention from members of AMREF's emergency team before being flown to hospital.

French team have had to contend with a difficult situation in a country riddled with problems. A woman doctor and three nurses started a mobile clinic. They travelled the length and breadth of the country, setting up in remote villages, administering antibiotics, cleaning up wounds, and generally doing all they could to help.

Mother Teresa

No history of nursing would be complete without a mention of Mother Teresa of Calcutta. Born in 1910 of Albanian parents at Skopje, Yugoslavia, she became a member of the Order of the Sisters of Our Lady of Loreto at the age of 18. She went to live in India and, after teaching for a time, obtained permission from her superior to live alone outside the cloister and to work among the poor in the Calcutta slums. In 1950 she received official approval for the establishment of a new congregation, the Missionaries of Charity, which subsequently began work in other parts of India and in many other countries, administering to the 'poorest of the poor' and bringing comfort to the sick and the dying.

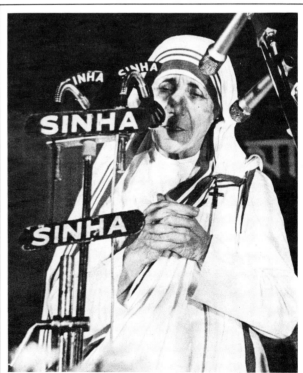

Mother Teresa addresses a crowd in Calcutta after being awarded the 1979 Nobel Peace Prize.

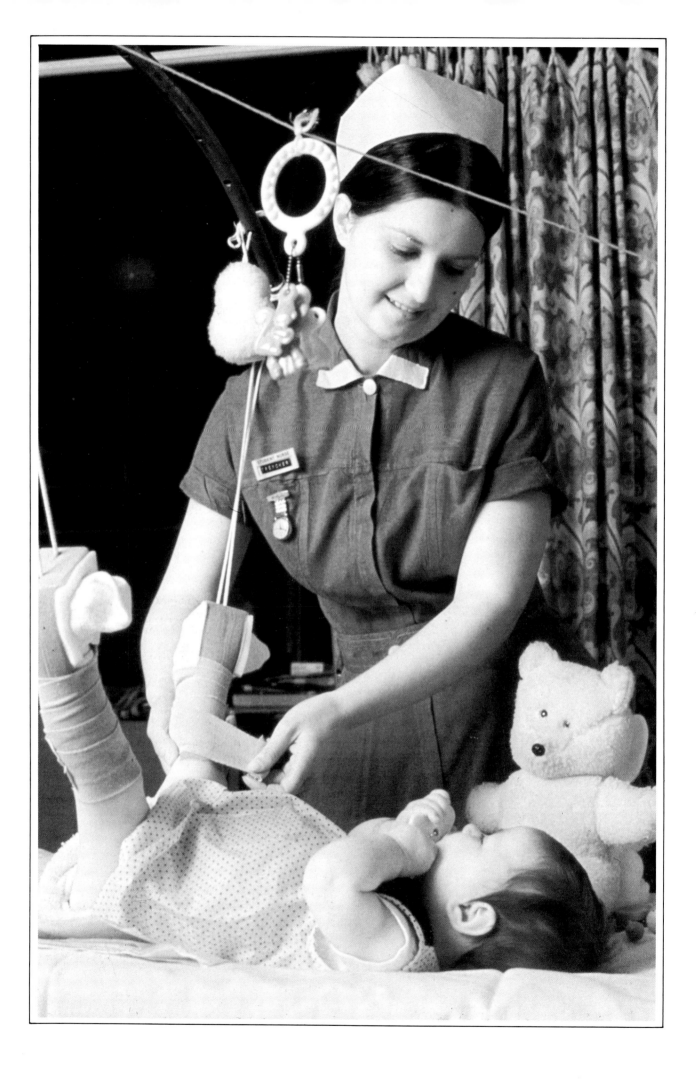

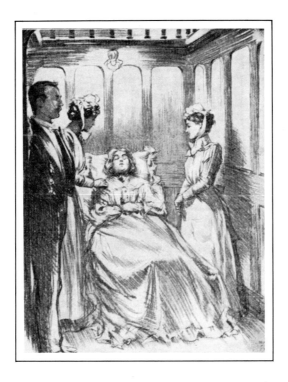

What is a nurse?

To the layman the fine building which houses the Royal College of Nursing is as much an institution as Broadcasting House, but many of its functions remain a mystery to the outsider. What is common knowledge, however, is that to be appointed general secretary of the College is a signal honour, and that those chosen to fill this demanding role must not only possess the necessary professional qualifications, experience and expertise, but must also have the highest principles, allied to qualities of leadership and diplomacy. The appointment of Dame Catherine Hall in 1957 proved to be both a wise and popular choice, and during the 25 years she spent as head of the College, she did much to help the nursing profession.

According to many senior nurses the pattern of nursing and the whole nature of hospital work have radically changed. New developments in anaesthetics, antibiotics and surgical techniques have widened the field of nursing considerably, and there are now many new fields open to nurses who wish to specialize. The National Health Service employs some 140,000 qualified nurses, with 76,000 in training. There are also many nurses employed outside the services and, although few work in private houses, many are to be found in private nursing homes and in industry and commerce.

Since the existence of patients is the sole justification for any system of nursing and medical care, it is interesting to note that until recently the role of the patient was a passive one. Even in this age the NHS patient, on entering hospital, still feels he is surrendering his identity when he surrenders his street clothes and, indeed, it is usually made clear to him from the beginning that 'his is not to reason why'. Patients are not supposed to ask questions about the state of their health.

However, efforts are being made to increase the nurse's awareness of the patient as a human being and also to prepare for her dealing with patients of different races and different cultures.

The lives of both patients and nurses, besides their common involvement with sickness, have other aspects which need to be taken into careful consideration. 'The sick, and those who care for them are simultaneously involved in intricate human relationships and associations which are of vital significance to the people concerned.'

The relationship between nurses and doctors has always been a complex one. So long as the role of the nurse was purely subjective, doctors felt secure, entrenched behind the bastions of their male-dominated universe. In general, the relationship between doctors and senior nurses ran comparatively smoothly, and the era of the starched, disciplined matron, waiting with shining morning smile to greet the surgeon or physician and accompanying him on his rounds was part of the traditional hospital pattern.

Today, however, the struggle to achieve equality between the sexes threatens to erode the long-established mores of the hospital staff, and the more militant and forceful the

Top *A specially enlarged lift in a private hospital in London in the early twentieth century. Illustration from* The Graphic, *17 June, 1903.*
Opposite *A nurse adjusting the traction and bandaging on the leg of a baby at Queen Mary's Hospital, Carshalton, Surrey.*

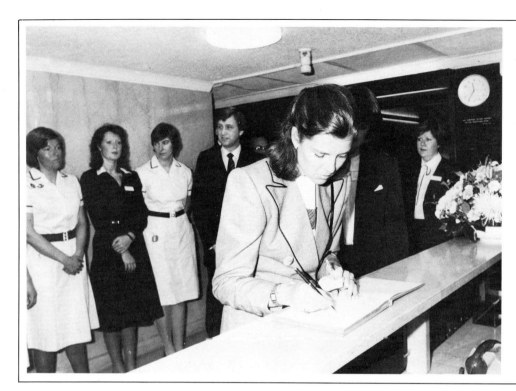

Princess Caroline of Monaco signs the visitor's book at the Princess Grace Hospital, London, in Oct. 1983. She opened the new intensive care unit at the hospital named after her mother.

feelings of the ardent feminists, the wider grows the gulf between nurse and doctor. Nor is the relationship between young doctors, male and female, and the mature, experienced senior nurses any smoother. It is to be hoped that the time is not far off when the right balance will be achieved between doctors and nurses, and both sexes will work in harmony, as a team, to the greater benefit of the patient.

At the quadrennial meeting of the International Council of Nurses held in Mexico in 1973, agreement was reached on the definition of a nurse, and on what constituted nursing.

> 'A nurse is a person who has completed a programme of basic nursing education and is qualified and authorized in his/her country to practice nursing. Basic nursing education is a formally recognized programme of study which provides a broad and sound foundation for the practice of nursing and for post-basic education which develops specific competence.'

> 'Nursing is concerned with caring for people throughout the span of life, and at all points on the continuum between sickness and health. Nursing is a profession in its own right. As such it has the right and responsibility to govern its own practice and professional affairs, and accepts a commitment to society in accordance with professional ethics.'

The need for a nursing service is universal, and the practice of nursing is unrestricted by nationality, race, colour, creed, age, sex, politics or social status. Nursing includes the promotion of health, the prevention of illness, the care of the sick, rehabilitation, and the care of the dying. It is practised in both institutional and non-institutional settings – in hospitals and in other premises provided specifically for health care services, in schools, in places of work and in people's own homes.

Nursing is concerned with the patient as a whole person and as a unique individual. The nurse respects the values, customs and spiritual beliefs of the individual, assesses and endeavours to meet his other nursing needs, and sees the individual within the context of the family, or other social unit, and within society as a whole. The nurse–patient relationship is a privileged one based on confidence (including confidentiality), trust and effective communication.

The three dimensions of nursing activity are clinical nursing practice, nursing education and the management of nursing services. These three functions are interdependent, of equal worth and share the common goal of the patient's well being.

The nurse of today has far wider horizons than before. She is no longer tied to a row of patients in a hospital ward. She can go out into the world, into the community of which she is so vital a part. She may be a district nurse attached to a general practice, a midwife or health visitor. She may nurse in a factory, prison, hospital ship, cruise liner, from a mobile clinic or in a disaster area. But, wherever she goes, she brings relief, order and a sense of security.

In her off-duty time, like her patients, she is affected by all the joys and sorrows of daily life but, once in her uniform, she is a link in the great chain of healing, a being apart. She is the archetypal woman, caring, gentle, and compassionate.

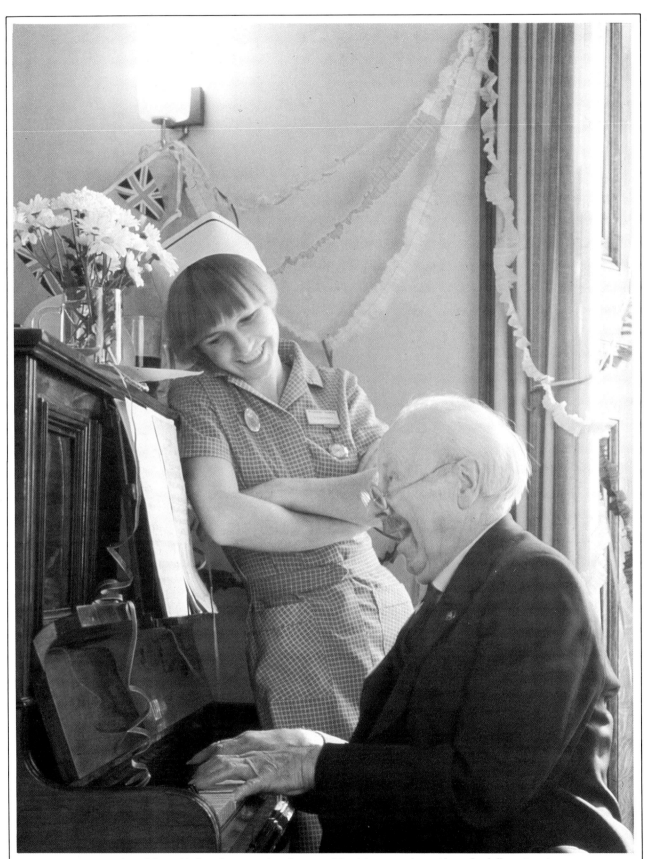

A nurse watches while an elderly male patient plays the piano. The ability to get along with people of all ages is an important quality in nursing.

Acknowledgments

The preparation of this book owes much to the works of so many specialists through the centuries that I should be hard pressed to enumerate them all. The *History of Medicine* was the original canvas on which I sketched in the history of nursing.

First and foremost on my lists of thanks is Ann Norman-Butler who, for many years, had a close association with the Royal College of Nursing. Without her patience, enthusiasm, knowledge and advice, this book might never have been completed. Without Ann I should not have made half the exciting discoveries of pictorial 'firsts' we found tucked away in institutions, libraries, museums and in private collections.

My most grateful thanks go to Trevor Clay, MPhil, SRN, RMN, the General Secretary of the Royal College of Nursing, both for his interest in this project and for his permission to consult the library of the Royal College of Nursing, which is one of the most complete in the world.

I also want to thank David Rye, BA, SRN, RMN, RNT, Director of Professional Activities at the Royal College of Nursing, for giving me some illuminating leads. I am also indebted to Monica Daly, an authority on the history of nursing, and Chairman of the RCN History of Nursing Group, for useful information.

I would like to thank the following for useful information and illustrations:
Royal Commonwealth Nursing Association – *Margaret Beard.*
Save the Children Fund – *Christopher Thornton and Diana Lacey.*
Princess Louise Children's Hospital, London.
African Medical and Research Foundation – *Elizabeth Young.*
Boer War National Army Museum, South Africa.
Women's Transport Service (First Aid Nursing Yeomanry) – *Major-General Charles Page, present Honorary Colonel.*
Women's Transport Service (First Aid Nursing Yeomanry) – *Miss Sheila Parkinson, present Commanding Officer.*
Professor Franco Crainz, MD, FRCOG.
Royal College of Midwives.
British Library – *Peter Jones, Department of Manuscripts.*
Victoria and Albert Museum – *Mrs Jennifer Opie, Department of Ceramics.*
Broadlands Archives – *Mrs Molly Chalk.*
Royal College of Obstetricians and Gynaecologists – *Patricia Want.*
Newcastle-upon-Tyne Polytechnic – *Kenneth McConkey.*
British Red Cross Society – *Miss M. N. Slade, Archivist.*
Queen Victoria Hospital, East Grinstead – *John Bennett.*
Princess Mary's Royal Air Force Nursing Service – *Wing Commander E.A.I. Sandison, ARRC, RNFAFNS.*
Royal Archives, Windsor Castle – *Elizabeth H. Cuthbert, Deputy Registrar.*
Wellcome Institute for the History of Nursing – *W. Schupbach.*
Wellcome Museum of the History of Medicine – *David Wright, Research.*
Commonwealth Nurses' Federation – *Miss M. A. Brayton.*
Catholic Missionary Society – *Miss M. Pavlovich, Secretary.*
South African Embassy, London – *R. Sheal.*
Chatsworth Settlement – *M. A. Pearman, Librarian.*
Royal College of Nursing – *Miss F. M. Walsh, Librarian.*
National Heart Hospital – *Dr Jane Somerville.*

Osborne House, Isle of Wight – *Surgeon Captain R. S. Macdonald,* MRCS, LRCP, DMRD, RN *(retd.), House Governor.*
Princess Grace Hospital, London (AMI Hospitals Ltd) – *Mrs Val Arnison.*
Fondation de France – *Lydie Veyret.*
Médecine du Monde, Paris.
Radcliffe College, Cambridge, Mass., USA – *Marie-Helene Gold.*
Charing Cross Hospital Medical School – *Howard Hagus.*
Missionary School of Medicine – *Mrs Jean Hayward-Lynch,* SRN, SCM.
British Film Institute – *Jenny Sussex.*
South African National Museum of Military History – *Col. George Duxbury.*
Ministry of Defence – *Second Officer P. G. Melville-Brown,* BA, WRNS, *Public Relations Officer* WRNS/QARNNS.
Queen Alexandra's Royal Naval Nursing Service – *Miss Jean Robertson, Matron-in-Chief.*
City Museum, Stoke-on-Trent – *Mrs K. Niblett, Assistant Keeper of Ceramics.*
The Order of St John Museum and Library – Miss Toffolo and Pamela Willis.
West Sussex Record Office – *Mrs Patricia Gill.*
Imperial War Museum.
British Association, Sovereign and Military Order of Malta – *David F. Bune, Vice-Chancellor.*
Mafeking Museum, South Africa – *Mrs Audrey Renew.*
Yale University Library, Beinecke Rare Book and Manuscript Library – *Julia B. Campbell.*
Yale University Medical Library, New Haven, Conn., USA.
McGill University, Montreal, Canada.
University of Pennsylvania, Philadelphia, USA – *Judie Malmudd.*
University of Virginia Library, Charlottesville, USA (Alderman Library) – *Janet R. Linde, Archivist.*
University of Louisville, USA – *Deborah Skaggs, Archivist. Sherrill McConnell, PhD, Archivist.*
Martin Gilliat, Private Secretary to Queen Elizabeth the Queen Mother, for information about Glamis Castle in wartime.
Madame Andrée de Jongh, GM.
Mrs Freda D. Siggins, Bermuda.
Bernard Price.
Ken Beal.
Vera Atkins.
Joan Atkins.
Dr Jack Penn, Capetown, South Africa.
Mrs Florence Dagg.
Susan Glen.
Joseph La Picirella, France.
Arthur Byron, France.
Viscount Norwich.
Their Graces the Duke and Duchess of Devonshire.
Countess Mountbatten of Burma.
Lady Pamela Hicks.
Sister Tutor Isobel Hancock.
Spink & Son Ltd – *A. R. Litherland, Medal Department.*
Colman's of Norwich – *M. H. Emanuel.*
Royal Worcester Spode Ltd – *Peter Croser.*

B. J. Boxall, *Chichester Health Authority.*
Josiah Wedgwood & Sons Ltd – *Mrs J. M. Bramfitt.*
Garrard & Co. Ltd – *A. Mann.*
Christie, Manson & Woods Ltd – *Peter Rose.*
Phillips Son & Neale – *James James-Cook.*
Sotheby's, London – *Michael Naxton, Department of Coins and Medals.*
Reckitt & Coleman Ltd.

I cannot omit the names of my friends who so valiantly answered my call and came up instantly with the addresses and information I required for my research. These include: the late and much regretted Doctor Thelma Gutsche; Karina Behr; Nicola Blundell Brown for useful contacts made during her world tour; Laurel Crosby and Juliet Mannock, Canada; Lady McIndoe and Paul Hanbury.

When I began collecting data for this work I had a notion that I was eventually going to write a history of nursing world-wide, and to this end I cast my net to the four corners of the globe. The response from archival sources, libraries, universities, hospitals, nursing colleges and nursing associations was prompt, exciting, fascinating and overwhelming, and, later, when I came to collate my material, preparatory to writing, I realized it would be an impossibility to include all the marvellous material sent me from the U.S.A., Canada, Australia, New Zealand, Bermuda, South America and Japan in one volume, particularly as the emphasis of my book was to be on its pictorial aspect rather than on its text.

I have, therefore, had perforce to confine myself, with some exceptions due to the specific nature of a particular chapter, to the history of nursing in the United Kingdom, but I have no doubt that the rich and invaluable lode of material lodged in my files will be gratefully tapped at some future date.

While I have collected, collated and examined all the material available to me on the history of nursing through the centuries, I want to state quite categorically that my conclusions and final summing up on the nature of nursing are entirely my own and, since I am a historian, are probably different from those of a nurse or a doctor.

I should be totally lacking in gratitude were I not to thank most warmly my assistant, Joan Hunt, whose work in connection with this book was above and beyond the call of duty; 'Tabby' who saw to it that I was free from hampering domestic chores; and Reg Davis-Poynter, whose advice and encouragement spurred me on.

No list of acknowledgements would be complete without thanking my friends in the West Sussex County Library, Chichester, who performed constant and tiny miracles in getting me the specialist literature I needed for my researches.

Bibliography

Brian Abel-Smith, *History of the Nursing Profession* (Heinemann, 1960)

P. Allan and M. Jolley (eds), *Nursing, Midwifery and Health Visiting since 1900* (Faber and Faber, 1982)

Enid Bagnold, *Autobiography* (Heinemann, 1969)

Monica E. Baly, *Nursing* (Batsford, 1977)

Stella Bingham, *Ministering Angels* (Osprey, 1979)

Gerald Bowman, *The Lamp and the Book* (Queen Anne Press, 1967)

C. J. Brim, *Medicine in the Bible* (Froben Press, New York, 1936)

Vera Brittain, *Testament of Youth* (Gollancz, 1978)

E. G. Browne, *Arabian Medicine* (Cambridge University Press, 1921)

J. M. Calder, *The Story of Nursing* (Methuen, 1955)

Arturo Castiglioni, *History of Medicine* (Alfred A. Knopf, New York, 1941)

Mary Chamberlain, *Old Wives' Tales* (Virago, 1981)

Alan Delgado, *As They Saw Her – Florence Nightingale* (Harrap, 1970)

I. E. Drabkin, *Medical Education in Greece and Rome* (London, 1944)

C. Elgood, *Medicine in Persia* (Hocher, New York, 1934)

J. Fisher, *That Miss Hobhouse* (Secker and Warburg, 1971)

H. Friedenwald, *The Jews and Medicine* (Johns Hopkins Press, New York, 1944)

E. Hagemann, *Ancient Egyptian Physicians* (London, 1926)

Margaret Hart, *Pre-Reformation Nurses in England* (John Murray, 1932)

Paul Hastings, *Medicine: An International History* (Ernest Benn, 1974)

H. W. Hoggard, *Mystery, Magic and Medicine* (Doubleday and Doran, New York, 1933)

M. J. Hughes, *Women Healers in Medieval Life and Literature* (King's Crown Press, New York, 1943)

Elspeth Huxley, *Florence Nightingale* (Chancellor Press, 1975)

Pat Jourdan, *District Nurse* (Weidenfeld and Nicolson, 1977)

H. K. Lewis, *Leper Houses and Medieval Hospitals* (London, 1915)

Elizabeth Longford, *Eminent Victorian Women* (Weidenfeld and Nicolson, 1981)

Brenda McBryde, *A Nurse's War* (Chatto and Windus, 1979)

Lynn MacDonald, *Roses of No Man's Land* (Michael Joseph, 1980)

Malcolm Muggeridge, *Something Beautiful for God* (Fontana, 1971)

D. G. Murphy, *They Did Not Pass By* (Longmans, 1956)

Beryl Oliver, *The British Red Cross In Action* (Faber, 1966)

Juliet Piggott, *Queen Alexandra's Royal Army Nursing Corps* (Leo Cooper, 1975)

J. H. Plumridge, *Hospital Ships and Ambulance Trains* (Seeley Service, 1975)

Evelyn Prentis, *A Nurse in Time* (Hutchinson, 1978)

D. Riesman, *The Story of Medicine in the Middle Ages* (Hoeber, New York, 1935)

June Rose, *Elizabeth Fry:* (Macmillan, 1980)

Rowland Ryder, *Edith Cavell* (Hamish Hamilton, 1975)

L. R. Seymer, *Florence Nightingale's Nurses* (Pitman Medical, 1960)

F. B. Smith, *Florence Nightingale: Reputation and Power* (Croom Helm, 1982)

Irene Ward, *F.A.N.Y. Invicta* (Hutchinson, 1955)

C. Woodham Smith, *Florence Nightingale, 1820–1910* (Constable, 1950)

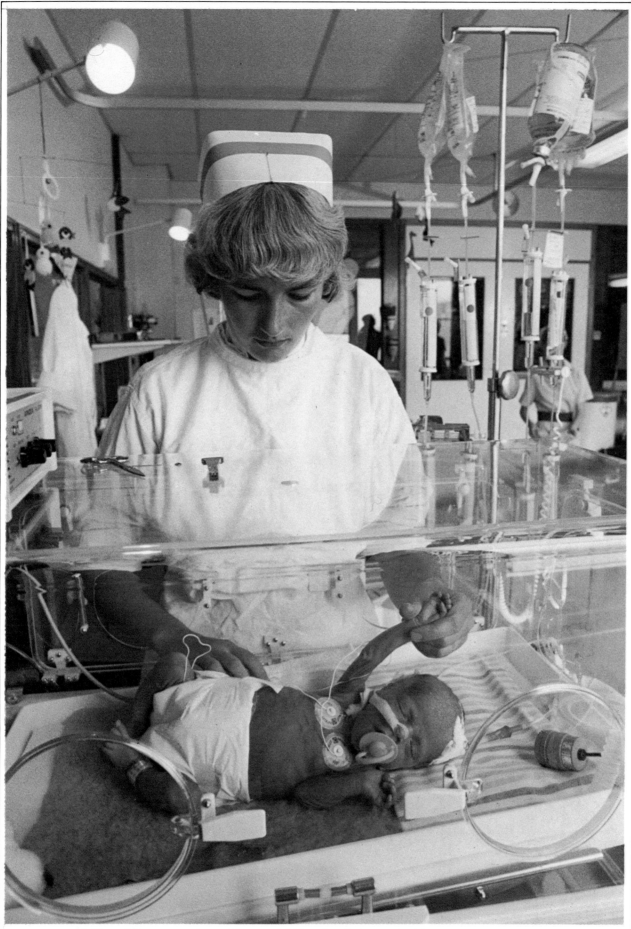

A nurse holding a baby in an incubator. The care of children from birth to early adolescence forms an important part of the post-registration courses for qualified state registered nurses.

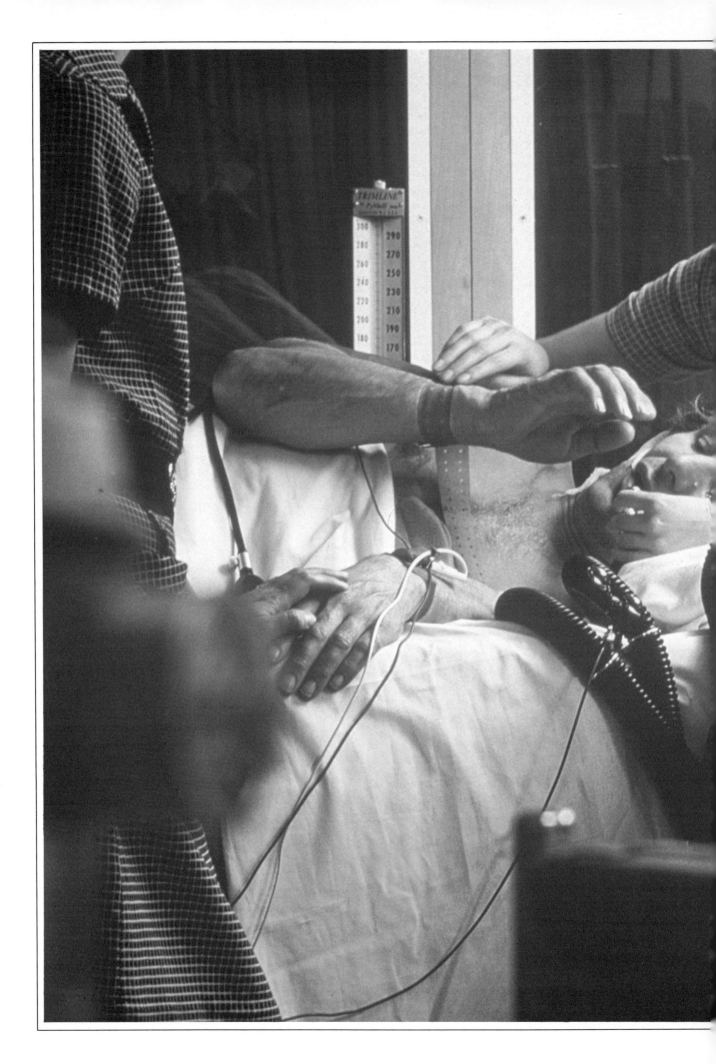

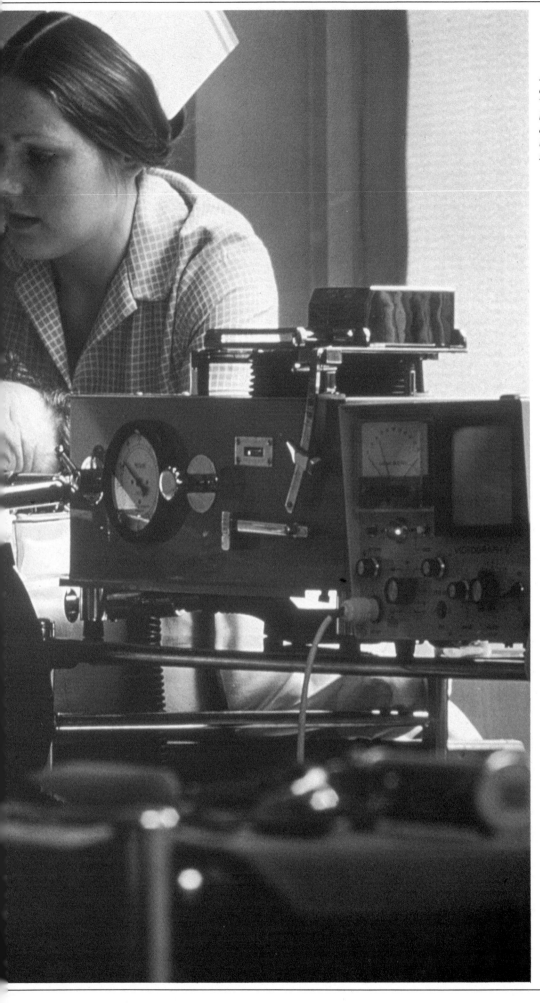

A patient receiving emergency treatment. The modern nurse must be able to cope with complex machinery and learn to develop special skills.

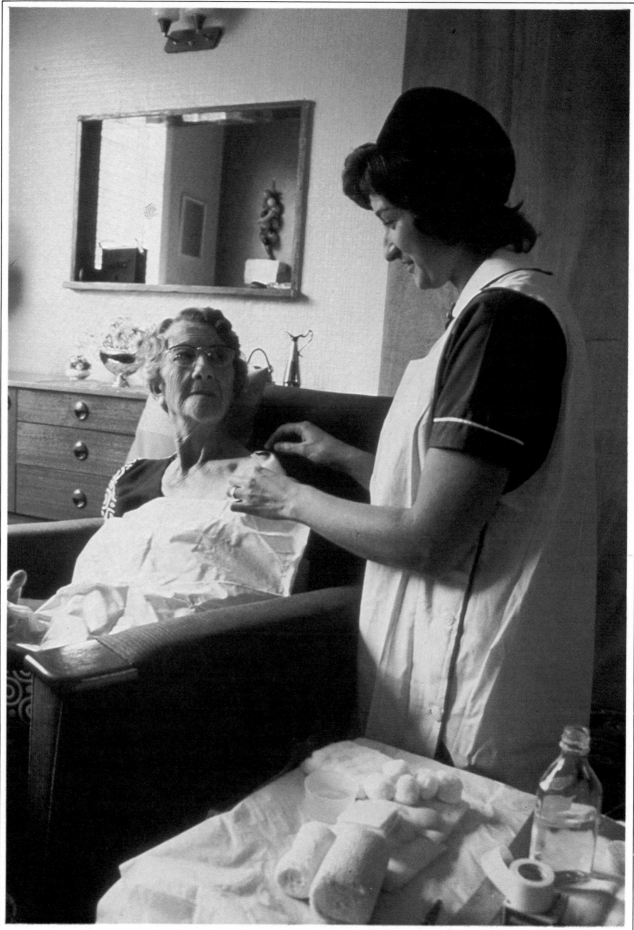

A nurse gives treatment to a patient at home. Since much more nursing is now being carried out in the home environment, the district nurse has a greater range of responsibilities.

Picture acknowledgments

The author and publishers wish to thank the following for their kind permission to reproduce illustrations contained in this book:

African Medical Research Foundation 157 top; AMI Hospitals Ltd 160; BBC Hulton Picture Library 10, 11, 12, 17 bottom, 18 left, 19, 22, 23, 24 right, 31, 32, 34 bottom, 40, 42, 45, 48, 49, 50, 51 left, 51 right, 52, 54, 60, 61, 62 top, 64, 70 top & bottom, 74 bottom, 77, 79, 82 bottom right, 94, 96 top & bottom, 97 bottom, 99, 103, 109, 110, 112 top, 113 top, 115 right, 121 bottom, 129, 130, 131, 133, 134 bottom, 139, 142, 143, 144, 146, 147 top, 147 bottom, 148, 150 top; Bettmann Archive, New York/BBC Hulton Picture Library 13 top, 14, 15 top, 20, 29, 33; Bodleian Library, Oxford 26 (MS. Douce 29, folio 23 verso), 27 (MS. Canon. Misc. 476, folio 27 detail), 28 (MS. Laud. Misc. 724, folio 97); The British Red Cross Society 80, 134 top right; Camera Press 149, 157 bottom/S. K. Dutt 152, 156; Central Office of Information 86, 87, 88, 125, 126–7, 128, 158, 161, 165, 166–7, 168; The Church Missionary Society/HGPL 154; The Imperial War Museum, London 85, 92 bottom, 102, 104, 105, 106, 108, 111 top & bottom, 112 bottom, 113 bottom, 114, 115 left, 121 top, 134 top left, 135, 136, 138, 140 right; The Mansell Collection 21, 35, 39, 46 bottom right, 75 top, 76, 78, 83, 89, 119, 153, 159; Mary Evans Picture Library 18 top & bottom right, 25, 30, 34 top, 37, 38 top, 53, 56, 58, 59, 65, 71 bottom, 75 bottom, 81, 97 top, 98; M. Masson 137; Ministry of Defence/Directorate of Public Relations (Navy) Photographic Department 84, 90/R.A.F. Department of Medical Photography 92 top; Musée de la Résistance du Vercors/J. La Picirella 140 left; The National Portrait Gallery, London 41, 55, 66; The Order of St John 82 top, 82 bottom left; The Royal College of Nursing Library 43, 67, 68, 116, 117, 122, 123, 124, 132, 145 bottom; Save the Children Fund/Mike Wells 155; The South African Nursing Association/Struik 95; Sotheby's, London 141; The University of Wales, College of Medicine 150 bottom.

B. T. Batsford Ltd for page 73 reproduced from M. Baly, *Nursing*. Struik/Cape Town for page 95 reproduced from C. Searle, *The History of the Development of Nursing in South Africa 1652–1960*.

Front cover: The Imperial War Museum, London.
Back cover: The Central Office of Information.
Frontispiece and endpapers: The BBC Hulton Picture Library.

Index